FIXING
YOUR FEET

**Preventative Maintenance and Treatments
for Foot Problems of Runners, Hikers,
and Adventure Racers**

FIXING
YOUR FEET

**Preventative Maintenance and Treatments
for Foot Problems of Runners, Hikers,
and Adventure Racers**

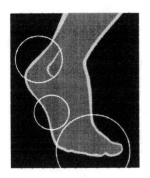

John Vonhof

WinePress Publishing 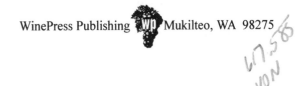 Mukilteo, WA 98275

PT

Copyright © 1997 by John Vonhof
Cover design copyright © 1997 by Kozak Design
Cover illustration copyright © 1997 by Adam Caldwell
Cover photographs copyright © 1997, Dan Campbell Photography (top two photos) and Gay Wiseman (bottom photo)
Illustrations copyright © 1997 by John Vonhof

Published by WinePress Publishing
PO Box 1406
Mukilteo, WA 98275

Printed in the United States of America

ISBN: 1-57921-026-0
Library of Congress Catalog Card Number: 97-060821

FIXING YOUR FEET
Preventative Maintenance and Treatments for Foot Problems of Runners, Hikers, and Adventure Racers.

Dedication

This book is first dedicated to my wife, Kathie, for her patience in the research and writing process and to my son, Scott, who gave me the idea after a 12-hour track run.

Secondly, this book is dedicated to the memory of my friend and ultrarunner, Dick Collins. Dick was the epitiome of what our sport needs: he was a good listener — always ready with encouragement, he was warm and sincere — taking honest pleasure in your success, he was always ready to lend a hand where needed — believing we should get involved in supporting and promoting our sports, and he loved the trails.

Acknowledgments

Thanks to Dr. Bill Trolan for reviewing the manuscript and providing his expertise and perspective as an emergency room physician, medical consulant to adventure racing teams, adventure racer, runner, hiker, and climber.

Thanks to Dennis Grandy, D.P.M. and David Hannaford, D.P.M. who reviewed the manuscript and provided valuable insights and advice from their podiatrist's perspective.

Thanks to Kirk Boisseree and Karl King for reviewing the manuscript.

Appreciation goes to Gary Cantrell and Suzi Thibeault (foot taping techniques), Andrew Lovy (lubricants), and Tom Crawford (skin tougheners), for their willingness to share what they have learned about how these factors affect foot care.

Thanks to *Ultrarunning* magazine for permission to reprint portions of Gary Cantrell's article, "From the South: The Amazing Miracle of Duct Tape," and Andrew Lovy's article, "New Blister Formula Revealed! Free!"

Contributors

Many thanks go to the following individuals who have contributed the tips and stories of what they have learned over the miles:

Ed Acheson
Steve Benjamin
Robert Boeder
Tony Burke
Dick Collins
Tom & Nancy Crawford
Valerie Doyle
Jay Hodde
Ivy Franklin
Ed Furtaw
Rob Grant
Karl King
Damon Lease
Andrew Lovy
Roy Pirrung
Dave Scott
Craig Smith
Frank Sutman
Dr. Bill Trolan
Will Uher
Nick Williams

Mike Bate
Richard Benyo
Kirk Boisseree
Gary Cantrell
Dave Covey
Orin Dahl
David Hannaford, D.P.M.
Andrew Ferguson
George Freelen
Dennis Grandy, D.P.M.
Matthew Jankowicz
Teresa Krall
Susie Lister
Matt Mahoney
Brick Robbins
Marv Skagerberg
Jillian Standish
Suzi Thibeault
Tim Twietmeyer
Paul Vorwerk

Foreword

Ever since our first ancestors stepped on the ground, we have been plagued by foot problems, especially blisters. Now they continue to afflict us in a variety of ways. You see them on hikers, runners, and athletic pursuits of all manner and description.

The last few years have seen the beginnings of adventure racing. I am fortunate to have been a part of this exciting new development in outdoor activity. The one factor that continues to amaze me is that individuals and teams will spend vast amounts of money, time, and thought on training, equipment, and travel, but little or no preparation on their feet. Too often the result has been that within a few hours to a few days all that work has been ruined. Ruined because the primary mode of transportation has broken down with blisters.

This problem is universal with hikers, runners, and any activity that requires feet. Most of these problems could easily be avoided with some preventative care. Other foot problems could have been taken care of with early treatment, stopping a small problem from becoming a costly one.

This book is the result of two years of research and writing. John has combed through hundreds of articles and reviewed previous literature on foot care. He has interviewed a multitude of people, many of them athletes who push the envelope of human endurance and passed their knowledge on to you. Further, he has reviewed hundreds of products all connected to preventing foot and blister problems. This wealth of information has been distilled down to this most comprehensive and extremely well written book.

This is it — the best book ever written on foot care! Everyone who has been bothered by foot problems or wants to prevent them should own this book. Its encyclopedic knowledge never ceases to amaze me. Despite having spent four years reading and taking care of blisters and other foot problems, every time I open this book I gain new information.

Billy Trolan, MD
Emergency Room Physician, author of the *Blister Fighter Guide,* and medical consulant to adventure racing teams.

Contents

Part Two: Preventative Maintenance

Part Three: Treatments

Introduction

In the world of running, problems with one's feet, whether in a 10K, a marathon, or an ultra, are the most common factors that prematurely end or ruin the run. Likewise, in the world of hiking, many a trip has been shortened because of blisters. Adventure racing, typically a unique multi-disciplined sport, requires healthy feet on all team participants at the same time, often over several days. One participant's bad feet can spell disaster for the whole team.

There are no shortcuts to finding what works for each of us. What works for one runner's feet may not work for another runner. The footcare efforts of one hiker or adventure racer may work wonders for him or her but cause you problems. This book offers information which has been tested by experienced runners, hikers, and adventure runners. If you study the information and make the application to your specific foot problems, by trial and error, you will determine what works for you. There are hundreds of tips in this book, but the bottom line is that you need to find which ones work for you. Try one. If it doesn't help, try another. Remember though, what works for you today may not work for you tomorrow and what works for me may not work for you.

By doing your homework, you'll be closer to solving your foot problems. If you are constantly plagued by blisters and use a lubricant, try powders; if you use cotton socks, try double layer socks; if you use moleskin, try one of the new blister patches. I recommend trying these fixes in your training, not during your competitive events or on your long-awaited hiking trip. Time spent learning what works for your feet can mean more time hiking or running and less time fixing problems when you don't want them or need them.

Two words sum up the advice in this book: *proactive* and *reactive*. Preventative maintenance is being *proactive* — working to solve problems before they develop. When problems develop, everything becomes *reactive* — working to solve an existing problem. Being *proactive* takes time up front. Being *reactive* takes time when you often do not have the time or the resources available and may put the event in jeopardy.

Some of you will read the material completely and make intelligent decisions about how to fix your feet. Educating yourself about preventative maintenance and implementing some of the ideas will help reduce your time spent treating problems. Others of you will skip right to the treatments section which describes the problem which you are now having without ever taking the time to read about and understand the components of preventative maintenance. You will very likely continue to have problems until you fully understand the importance of *proactive* prevention before *reactive* treatment.

The real eye-opener, as I researched material and interviewed athletes for the book was:

☞ the extent of the problems so many athletes have with their feet;
☞ that so many of these same athletes naturally expect to have problems, because;
☞ what has worked for them in the past no longer works;
☞ what they see other athletes do with their feet does not work for them, and;
☞ they do not know what options they have to fix their feet.

This eye-opener led me to: research related books, articles, medical studies; contact numerous companies about their products and services and what they could do for our feet; consult with medical specialists; and talk to runners, hikers, and adventure racers. What I envisioned as a short booklet quickly turned into a book. My office swelled with stacks of product brochures, books, magazines, and boxes of sample products. Encouraged by those I talked to, the project grew.

Dennis Grandy, D.P.M., the Western States 100 Mile Endurance Run Podiatry Director, has treated the foot problems of many hundreds of runners. He has seen "... many conditions that were treated 'on the spot' with no medical reference ever being available. Blisters, although very common, are usually overlooked and often cause the runner to drop from the race." David Hannaford, D.P.M, is a sports podiatrist to many Olympians, ultrarunners, and other endurance athletes. Dr. Bill Trolan has served as medical consulant to adventure racing teams, fixing many participant's feet. Each of these doctors has treated many, many athletes whose runs, hikes, and adventure races are jeopardized because of foot problems. Their experiences underscore the need for this book about *Fixing Your Feet*.

Dave Scott, a good friend and very capable ultrarunner, put the foot problem in proper perspective when he said "When you don't take care of your feet during a long run or race, each step becomes a reminder of your ignorance." My goal in writing this book is to give you the information necessary to make informed and intelligent choices in both the prevention and treatment of your foot problems.

Whether you are a 10 km runner, a marathoner, or an ultrarunner; an overnight hiker or a long-distance thru-hiker; or a novice or veteran multi-sport adventure racer, this book can help you understand how to keep your feet healthy.

This book contains numerous references to products and services but makes no judgment call about the products or about one product being better than another. I have listed these products in alphabetical order for the sake of simplicity. The order does not imply one product is more helpful or less helpful than another.

Part One

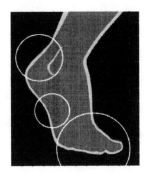

The Basics

1

Seeking Medical Treatment

The information and advice given in this book is provided to runners, hikers, and adventure racers to use in their effort to resolve foot problems. Not all foot problems or injuries will be resolved successfully by following the tips mentioned in this book.

Never ignore an injury. Pushing through an injury or returning to your sport too early after being injured can lead to additional injuries. You do not want to turn a temporary injury into a permanent disability.

If you have persistent foot problems or recurring pain during or after running or hiking which you cannot resolve, you are advised to seek medical treatment from a medical specialist who can provide his or her medical expertise for your problem. The two main medical specialists for the feet are:

☞ orthopedic surgeons, commonly called *orthopedists*, are experts for the joints, muscles and bones. This includes your knees, legs, pelvis, and spine. Look for an orthopedist who specializes in the foot and ankle.

☞ podiatrists are experts who work on the feet up to and including the ankles.

There is a wide range of skill overlap between orthopedists and podiatrists. Each can treat most of the same foot problems. Talk to them about their training, experience, and whether they have a specialty field. Weigh this information when making a decision about who to turn to for help.

Listen to your whole body and especially your feet. Be attentive to when the pain begins and what makes it hurt more or less. Be prepared to tell the specialist about the problem, its history, what you have done to correct it, and whether it worked or got worse. When the time comes to seek medical attention, ask others in your sport for referrals or look in the Yellow Pages. If you have a choice, choose a sports medicine specialist over a general doctor. The American Academy of Podiatric Sports Medicine, the American Academy of Orthopaedic Surgeons, and the American Orthopaedic Foot and Ankle Society can provide information and referrals. See the chapter *Medical Specialists* on page 157 for their telephone numbers.

2

Running, Hiking, Adventure Racing, and Your Feet

The physically taxing acts of running, hiking, and adventure racing place extreme demands on our feet. And in each sport there are wide ranges of difficulty. Where else are our feet forced to put up with such stresses in often adverse conditions?

Running may be a relatively short road 10 km or a grueling ultrarunning event of 100 miles with over 40,000 feet of mountainous ascents and descents. There are also further extremes: 24-, 48-, and 72-hour runs, six-day runs, and 1000-mile races. The terrain may be paved roads, tracks, fire roads, trails, or cross-country. You may run without any gear, with a single water bottle, or carry a fanny pack loaded with extra socks, food, and waterbottles.

Hiking may be a day trip with a day pack, an overnighter with a mid-weight 40-pound backpack, or a ten-day high-Sierra trip with a pack which tips the scales at 65 pounds. You may be a regular-style backpacker with a full-size pack which carries all the comforts of home. Or you may be a fastpacker with a 30-pound pack or an ultralight backpacker with a 20-pound pack. Regular backpackers may cover six to ten miles in a day, fastpackers may cover 20 miles, while ultralight backpackers can easily cover 30 miles or more. The hike may be an overnighter in your local hills, a week in the desert, a three-week backpack in the Sierras, or a several month thru-hike on the Appalachian Trail or the Pacific Crest Trail.

Adventure racing includes events with names like Eco-Challenge®, the Raid Gauloises, or the Extreme Games. These are typically competitive team races with up to five participants who must all finish together. With a combination of sports disciplines like trail or cross-country running, mountain biking, rappelling, climbing, kayaking, canoeing, horse back riding, swimming, glacier climbing, and others, the challenge is an often unknown course with constantly changing terrain. Many are multi-day events over distances up to 300 miles. Paging through several sporting publications I found several of these events advertised: the "Hi-Tec Adventure Racing Series," the first nationwide adventure racing series; "The Longest Day Adventure Race," a 32-hour, 100 mile, seven discipline event; the "Eco-Challenge Race Series," a fast-paced, two-day event; and the "Four Winds Adventure Race," a 300-mile, six discipline event. Additionally, individuals experienced in these events are offering training schools to instruct "would-be" adventure racers in the finer points of success across the sport disciplines.

What do these sports have in common? They pound, stress, and strain our feet to often unnatural extremes while causing problems and injuries. Proper foot care is the most important variable for a successful outing.

Sport Similarities

The similarities between the three sports are numerous. All three sports:
☞ pound the feet, stress the joints, and strain the muscles
☞ may be done in a day's time, yet often are done over several days, or even a week or more
☞ make the feet highly susceptible to hot spots, blisters, and problems with toenails, stubbed toes, bruises, sprains, strains, heels spurs, plantar fasciitis, and Achilles tendinitis
☞ can be enjoyed more by solving these common foot problems

While hikers move slower than runners, the weight of a fully loaded fannypack, lumbar pack, or backpack can easily stress the feet just as the weight a runner places on his or her feet. Adventure racers may stress the feet faster in shorter events and longer over multi-day events because of added stresses from the multi-sport multi-day events because of added stresses from the multi-sport disciplines and/or the special equipment they may have to carry. The longer multi-day adventure races often tax the feet more than we can imagine with their constant exposure to water or constantly changing adverse conditions.

Studies have shown that "Carrying heavy external loads, (e.g. a heavy backpack) during locomotion appears to increase the likelihood of foot blisters."[1] In addition, the type of physical activity performed is a factor in the probability of blister development. As we intensify our activity and as the duration of the activity increases, frictional forces are increased. Heavy loads, high-intensity activities, and long duration activities describe what we do as runners, hikers, and adventure racers. Most of us perform at least two of these three activities. Ultrarunner Suzie Lister typically experiences few problems with her feet while running ultras. However, when she participated in the 1995 Eco-Challenge the added weight of a pack on her back and the multi-day stresses of adventure racing caused many problems with her feet: blisters-on-top-of-blisters and swollen feet.

The similarities in the three sports make the preventative maintenance and treatments for blisters and other foot problems work for all three. The book approaches the different disciplines: running, hiking, and adventure racing, as one-and-the-same when dealing with one's feet.

3

Biomechanics

Biomechanics is the study of the mechanics of a living body, especially of the forces exerted by muscles and gravity on the skeletal structure. The foot, which includes everything below the ankle, is a complicated but amazing structure. With 26 bones each, together they account for almost one-quarter the total number of bones in the

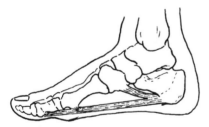

Side view of the bones of foot

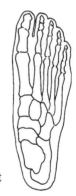

Top view of the bones of the foot

entire body. There are thirty-three joints to make the feet flexible. Control of the foot's movements is managed by about 20 muscles. Tendons stretch like rubber bands between the bones and muscles so that when a muscle contracts, the tendon pulls the bone. Each foot contains more than 100 ligaments which connect bone to bone and cartilage to bone and hold the whole structure together. Nerve endings make the feet sensitive. With each step you walk or run, your feet are subjected to a force of two to three times your body weight, which makes the feet prone to injury.

The big toe, commonly called the *great toe*, helps to maintain balance while the little toes function like a springboard. The three inner metatarsal bones provide rigid support while the two outer metatarsal bones, one on each side of the foot, move to adapt to uneven surfaces.

Your feet are each supported by two arches. The transverse arch runs from side-to-side just back from the ball of the foot. This is the major weight-bearing arch of the foot. The medial longitudinal arch runs the length of the instep, flattening while standing or running and shortening when you sit or lie down, giving spring to the gait. The lateral longitudinal arch runs on the outside of the foot.

Transverse arch

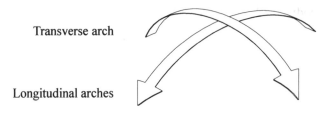

Longitudinal arches

Both longitudinal arches function in absorbing shock loads and balancing the body. These three arches of the foot are referred to singularly as the foot's arch.

The body lines up over the foot. When the foot goes out of alignment, the ankle, knee, pelvis, and back may all follow. Analyzing the way we stand, walk, and run helps a podiatrist or orthopedist determine whether we have a mechanical misalignment and how it can be corrected. He or she will also want to see your running shoes to analyze the wear patterns on the soles.

An example of biomechanics is how the foot's arch works. A low arch, or flat foot, typically occurs when the foot is excessively pronated, turning it inward. A high arch supinates the foot, rolling it outward. Both of these structural variations can cause knee, hip, and back pain. When one arch flattens more than the other arch, that inner ankle moves closer to the ground. That hip then rotates downward and backward causing a shortening of that leg during walking and running. The pelvis and back both tilt lower on the shortened leg side and the back bends sideways. The opposite leg, which is now longer, is moved outward towards the side which puts added stress on its ankle, knee, and hip. The shoulder on that side then drops towards the dropped hip. All of these are compensations as the body adapts. Muscles, tendons, ligaments and joints are stretched to their limit. The body is out of alignment.

The stresses on our bodies can result in inflammation, often the cause of foot pain. Running on unbalanced and uneven feet may result in fatigue. Fatigue gives way to spasms which may cause a shift in the shape of our feet. Corns, calluses, bunions, spurs, and neuromas may develop when joints are out of alignment.

Do not fall into the trap of drawing erroneous conclusions about your injuries or the type of shoes or equipment you need for your running style. Pain associated with running should be checked by a podiatrist or orthopedist. Heel pain that we try to resolve with a heel pad may not be caused by a heel problem, but by arch problems. This in turn may throw off the biomechanics of the body's alignment. If you begin a run and right away experience knee pain, you most likely have a problem with the knee. If the pain comes after running for a while, it is most likely not a knee problem but a biomechanical problem. Likewise, you may think because you are a heavy runner you need a shoe with lots of cushioning. Based on that decision, you buy a cushioned shoe, the most cushioning insoles, and wear thickly cushioned socks. But, in reality, what you may need is a stability control shoe. This is where the help and expertise of medical specialists comes in. They are trained to determine biomechanical problems.

In 1991, Craig Smith and his brother set out to hike 300 miles of the Continental Divide Trail. With training and planning done, they started with heavy packs which tipped the scale at almost 58 pounds each. Two days and twenty-two miles later Craig had developed severe pain in both knees. Forced to abort the trip, they cached as much gear as possible before starting back. With Craig's knees wrapped with torn T-shirt strips, it took them four days to backtrack the twenty-two miles. It took several weeks of conditioning therapy before he could finally walk without a limp. Craig now packs lighter, does exercises that focus on strengthening the knees, and uses a walking stick on downhills. He could have easily been a victim of biomechanical problems which centered in his knees.

Remember that most athletes have foot problems or become injured by doing too much, too soon, too fast. To avoid biomechanical problems, use proper footwear, pace yourself, and do strength training.

4

Where You Run and Hike

The terrain is an important part of your running and hiking environment. While a flat, smooth, and resilient surface is ideal, most of us do not have that luxury. Nor do many of us want that type of surface. Most runners spend the majority of their running miles on roads while most hikers spend their time on trails. Variations from our normal running surface can produce problems as we compensate for uphills, downhills, concave surfaces, or irregularities of the surface.

Sidewalks

Concrete sidewalks are harder than any other surface for running. This surface can cause foot, leg or back pain through the jarring of the joints. Care must be taken to watch your footing on sidewalks to avoid the tapered edges of driveways and drop-offs at curbs.

Roads

Road running is the mainstay of most runners. The asphalt surface of most roads provides a softer surface than concrete sidewalks. The problem with roads is the slanted, concave surface curving down towards the sides. Spend a few minutes on your favorite roads to see the angle of their curve and be aware of it. The concave surface puts more stress on the downward side of your shoes and your body. The foot of the higher leg rotates inward while the foot of the lower leg rotates outward and acts as a shortened leg. Avoid prolonged running on slanted surfaces. Keep your eyes open for potholes and manhole covers. Of course, the biggest hazard to road runners is vehicles. Where possible, run opposite the flow of traffic and safely to one side of the road.

Trails

Trails provide a soft running and hiking surface. Trail running, whether on single-track trails or fire roads, can open new vistas to the adventuresome runner. Whether running or hiking, care must be taken to pay close attention to trail hazards like rocks, roots, wet leaves, mud, etc., all of which can cause a turned ankle or a fall. Trail dust, dirt, pebbles, and rocks can be kicked up into the sock or between the sock and the shoe. These irritants can cause hot spots, blisters, or cuts. Gaiters worn over the shoe or boot tops can help prevent this problem. On rainy days, slippery mud and grasses can present problems with footing. On the occasional grassy sections of trail watch for uneven terrain and holes.

Hiking on trails while wearing a full backpack presents the added problem of maintaining one's balance with a top-heavy load while negotiating rocks, roots, and uneven trail. Attention to your footing, along with supportive boots, can help prevent a turned ankle. Uphills stretch the Achilles tendons, the calf muscles, and makes the pelvis tilt forward. Downhills increases the impact shock to the heel when landing and tilts the body backward. Continued up-hills and down-hills may also cause problems with toes, toenails, heel pain, plantar fasciitis, and more.

Tracks

Most runners, at some time, run on tracks. True, they can be boring. Running in circles, actually in ovals, lap after lap after lap after lap may not be your idea of a good run, but there may be a time for it in your running schedule. A track allows us to find out with accuracy how fast we are running. I have used a track for occasional speed workouts. Prior to my first 24-hour track run, I spent three hours running at a local high-school track to "get a feel" for the repetiveness of track running. The continuous running in one direction stresses the outer leg, so change direction every now and then. Dirt tracks should always be checked for ruts and uneven surfaces which could cause you to trip.

5

Running Shoes, Boots, Sandals, and Insoles

Running and hiking, as far as the feet go, require very little basic equipment. The basics are shoes or boots, socks, and insoles. Yet the war against foot problems can be lost over ill-fitting shoes or boots, socks which cause blisters, or insoles which are not right for your activity. This chapter focuses on running shoes, hiking boots, getting a good fit, and insoles. Sandals are briefly discussed because they are becoming popular. Because socks play such a large role in preventative maintenance, they are discussed at length in the next chapter.

Our feet are unique. Yours may look similar to mine, yet they are as different as our fingerprints. Although our feet may fit into the same size and shape of shoe or boot, there are differences in how our feet actually mold into the shoe. Corns, bunions, susceptibility to blisters, toe length, the type of arches, and the shape of our feet are just a few of the factors which affect our fit into shoes. Even how we react to and recover from the stresses of running and hiking is important to choosing shoes and boots.

Only you can determine what type of footwear you need to wear. Certainly runners wear running shoes, but there are many types of running shoes. Hikers and adventure racers have many choices in hiking boots but many make the choice to wear running shoes instead of boots. Many of the top teams racing the 1996 Eco-Challenge wore running shoes for the whole event, even on snow and ice and while wearing crampons. Just remember the "ifs." If you are used to hiking in running shoes, if your ankles are strong, and if the shoes provide the necessary support while wearing a pack, then running shoes may be right for you. Choose your footwear based on which sport you will be doing, the terrain expected, and your level of experience.

Whether wearing running shoes or boots, remember to inspect them regularly for problems. Frank Sutman was on the second day of a six-day 80-mile backpack trip when one of his boot's outersole split from the midsole to the ball of the foot. He suffered through four days of flapping sole, picking up pebbles, rocks, sticks, and even being tripped up. The moral of his story is to check your boots and shoes before major activities and periodically to keep small problems from becoming major inconveniences. Split outersoles, ripped or torn fabric which lets dirt and rocks into the shoe, cracked heel counters which create folds in the inner heel material, or broken laces retied into a bothersome knot over the top of the foot are all preventable.

Running Shoes

There are many sources of information about which shoes may be the best for you. The five main sources are the shoe companies, local running stores, running magazines, running catalogs, and running friends. Recognize the difference in the quality of help available from some "chain" shoe stores in shopping malls and that from a store which specializes in running shoes and equipment. A specialized running store usually has personnel who are runners themselves and can watch you run, look at your old shoes, and recommend specific brands of shoes and styles based on what they see and your answers to their questions.

The form over which a shoe or boot is constructed is called a last. Running shoes are built on one of several last patterns.

☞ Board last shoes have the shoe's upper material glued to the shoe's board, which runs the length of the shoe. This generally produces a fairly rigid and stable shoe.

☞ Combination last shoes have the shoe's upper material stitched to either the forefoot (slip-lasted) or the rearfoot (board-lasted). This design offers additional stability at either the footplant or the toe's push-off.

☞ Semicurved lasts are molded straight towards the rearfoot while having some curve towards the forefoot. This mold provides stability and flexibility.

☞ Semistraight lasts are built to curve slightly from the toe to the heel. This provides some flexibility and a high degree of stability.

☞ Straight last shoes are built along the shoe's straight arch to provide maximum stability.

☞ Slip last shoes are made with the upper material stitched directly to the midsole without a board. This offers maximum flexibility.

Running shoes can be grouped into several categories.

☞ Neutral shoes are made for the runner who has good biomechanics and would be categorized as a neutral pronator. These shoes generally have a good blend of flexibility and stability.

☞ Flexibility shoes are made for runners who are under-pronators, with foot motion towards the outside and who need a shoe which offers more shock-absorbing pronation than their body delivers.

☞ Stability shoes offer high stability and cushioning. These are typically used by mid-weight or normal arched runners without motion problems who are looking for good cushioning. These runners usually over-pronate slightly beyond neutral and need a shoe with extra medial support. Most are built on a semicurved last.

☞ Motion-control shoes are those which provide the most control, rigidity, and stability. These are often used by heavy runners, severe over-pronators, flat feet runners, and orthotic users. They are typically quite durable shoes but often at a cost of being heavier. Most are built on a straight last and offer the greatest level of medial support.

☞ Trail running shoes are those which usually offer increased toe protection, outersole traction, stability, and durability. These are usually used by runners who run mainly on trails.

☞ Cushioned shoes are simply those with the best cushioning. These are typically used by those who do not need extra medial support and by high-arched runners. Most are built on a curved or semicurved last.

☞ Lightweight shoes are those typically made for fast training or racing. These come with varying degrees of stability and cushioning and can be worn by runners with little or no foot problems. Most are built on a curved or semicurved last.

Shoe designs are always changing. Often our favorite shoes disappear from the shelves and we find ourselves forced to make new choices. Do your homework, study the shoe reviews and the ads, talk to your running friends, and try them on. Good stores will let you run in them. Orin Dahl once found that his favorite shoes were no longer offered. Instead of the old shoes, Nike offered a new type of "air" shoe. He bought the shoes and began running in them. The new shoes were not as flexible in the forefoot which caused his heel to pull up and out of the shoe. To his dismay, he developed blisters at the back of his heels. He recalls how he turned the shoes over to the Salvation Army and began a search for a different pair. He has no doubt that the shoes were good shoes. They were just not right for his feet and running style. As you look for shoes, remember that not every pair of shoes is right for your feet.

Hiking Boots

My first pair of hiking boots were all leather, with thick Virbram® soles, laced all the way to my calf, and seemed to weigh as much as my loaded backpack. Times have changed and so have hiking boots. Because of technology, they fit better and are easier on your feet. Running shoe technology has had a positive influence on hiking boots. Insoles, molding, padding, and midsole and outersole advances have made many of them as comfortable as lighter-weight boots.

Many hikers have been converted to using the newer lightweight boots. These are usually as flexible as running shoes and carry many of the running shoe benefits of fit and comfort. Because of their flexibility and construction, many of these require very little or no break-in time. I completed an 8.5-day, 221-mile ultra-light backpack of the John Muir Trail in regular running shoes. Unless you are used to hiking or running trails in running shoes while wearing a backpack, I do not recommend them for backpacking. Since I did the John Muir Trail in 1987, boots have changed. Today, I would consider a trail running shoe or lightweight boot for the same hike.

Check out some of the features of new hiking boots at your local store. Many boots offer a combination of features: lighter weight, breathable uppers, high-traction and long-lasting outsoles, improved lacing systems, flexible footbeds, stable and cushioning midsoles, wider toe boxes, and Gore-Tex® fabric incorporated into the uppers. Boots can be rated in three categories: lightweight hiking — for trail hiking and light loads; midweight hiking — for on/off trail hiking and light backpacking; and heavyweight hiking — for on/off trail, heavy loads, and multi-day trips. First, determine the type of hiking you will be doing and how much support and protection you will need for the weight you will carry. Second, look at the various features of different boots in each of the three categories. Then shop accordingly, but do not rule out a certain type of boot until you try them on your feet. Remember, a boot that pinches or rubs in the store will not feel better when you are out on the trail.

Before buying boots, check *Backpacker* and *Outside* magazines for their coverage on hiking boots. These articles evaluate most brands based on fixed standards while identifying their features and costs. Then check out your local backpacking supply store for the brands and styles they carry. Spend as much time as is necessary to get a good fit. Tell the salesperson what type of hiking you will be doing, for how long, and how much weight you plan on carrying. Try on several pairs of boots by different companies. Use your own socks. Put a weighted pack on your back if possible. Walk in the boots. Squat in them. Look for a pair that fits right from the start and grips your heels. Take out the insoles and look at the boot's construction. Find the pair that fits and feels better than the others. Purchase a high-quality boot made for hiking rather than lightweight boots sold for general street wear. These "fashion-statement" boots will not hold up under the stresses of heavy trail use. Utilize the experience of the personnel of your local camping and backpacking stores to help you in making a wise decision, but realize the final decision is yours based on how they feel on your feet.

Remember that the boots you select will each be picked up and put down many times each day. Hiking 12 miles each day would equate to 25,000 steps[2], day after day. Feel the weight of your boot and think about each step. Heavier boots are not always the best. True, they may provide more ankle stabilization, but you could get more benefit from a lightweight boot and proper ankle and foot strength conditioning before the hike. Ray Jardine, who has hiked the Pacific Crest Trail three times and the Appalachian and Continental Divide Trails each once, estimates that each 3.5 ounces off a pair of boots will add about a mile to a day's hiking progress.[3] A review of one store's boot selection showed weights for a pair of boots ranging from one pound nine ounces all the way to three pounds nine ounces. Selecting boots that weigh 10.5 ounces less than another pair could mean an additional three miles hiked per day. An educated choice, based on boot features, your personal needs, and the terrain ahead is necessary.

Ed Acheson made several painful discoveries when he hiked the Pacific Crest Trail. With his boots not completely broken in, he switched to a different pair on a salesperson's recommendation. The boots were too much boot for him and a half size too small — the salesperson told him they were sized larger than most. Ed remembers for the first 20 days having "... more blisters than the number of days I had been out." Because of the blisters he compensated his gait which in turn gave him knee problems. Before he could get new boots he was forced to cross the Mojave in tennis shoes. He still suffers from problems he attributes to the wrong boots.

If you are planning a several-week hike or a several-month thru-hike on a multi-state trail, remember the need to buy boots larger than normal to accommodate your feet as they become stronger and enlarge to their normal hiking size. Try on boots that are anywhere from one to two sizes larger than normal, which will allow your feet to fit into them properly.

Some boots will soften and become more flexible with forceful flexion of the soles and uppers, hand-working of waterproofing solution into the leather, or mechanical flexion of the uppers at a shoe shop. If your boots are too stiff try one of these three methods.

A week into hiking the John Muir Trail, Andrew Ferguson developed a "hellatious" deep blister on the back of his right foot, about 1.5″ in diameter. By nursing the blister with Spenco 2nd Skin and tape he hiked for three days in running shoes before reaching civilization and purchasing a new pair of boots. The red heel bothered him for two weeks and took six months to return to normal. Andrew is now a believer in running shoes for hiking. Many people prefer running shoes instead of boots for hiking.

If you are always having problems with your boots and a different set of boots does not help, consider trying a pair of running shoes, preferably trail running shoes. Be aware, however, of the differences. Running shoes do not provide the same degree of ankle support and overall foot protection. While some may prefer the increased ankle mobility in a low running shoe, this choice requires proper strength in the feet, ankles, and legs. My choice to wear running shoes when fastpacking the 221 miles of the John Muir Trail was based on a trial overnight hike with a full backpack and years of running trails. I knew my feet and ankles could handle the stresses of the trail in running shoes and I did not need heavier boots.

When you do have problems with your feet, and you usually will at some point, you need to look at the boots and evaluate whether you need to replace them with another boot type and/or style. On long hikes, your feet do enlarge and change. Boots wear out. Over a couple of years your feet may also change. Be open to new styles and features in newer type boots and find the pair that best fits you.

Sandals

Sandals are becoming more popular as designs improve to provide better traction, foot control, and comfort. Changing from running shoes or hiking boots into an open pair of sandals can be refreshing. When your feet are tired, hot, or sore, sandals can feel like a small piece of heaven on earth.

When shopping for sandals, try several designs. The straps may rub you wrong. A different style may offer straps that fit better. Some strapping systems require readjustment each time you put them on. If you will be wearing socks with them, be sure they have adequate space for your socks. Look at the soles for adequate traction design. Some designs offer a lip around the edge of the sandal which can provide a degree of protection from rocks and roots.

Wearing sandals while running or hiking takes getting used to. Small pebbles, gravel, leaves, or other debris can easily work their way underfoot. Shaking the foot or a light kick against a rock will usually knock these loose. Be especially careful of sticks on the trail which could inflict a puncture wound to your exposed feet. If you wear sandals without socks the skin of the foot will eventually toughen into calluses. Check the calluses regularly for cracks which can split through to uncalloused skin and bleed or become infected.

Tired of running shoes that fit him poorly, caused blisters and toenail problems, and seemed to collect dirt, Rob Grant bought a pair of sandals. He used his Teva Terradactyls in a Sri Chinmoy 24-Hour Run. At 100 km both small toes were swollen. The next day he ground down the ridge on the footbeds which fits under the toes. This corrected the problem. After putting 405 miles on the sandals, he reports no noticeable wear on the soles or the straps. Rob found that rubbing Vaseline on the inside of the straps helped to soften then when first used. He feels that ankle support in sandals is comparable to that of running shoes.

Getting a Proper Fit

Many shoe and boot companies suggest which of their models are best for certain types of activities, certain types of feet, and certain types of runners or hikers. Look for the *Runner's World* shoe-buyer's guides, the *Running Times* shoe reviews, *Backpacking* magazine's boot reviews, and *Outside* magazine's Buyer's Guide for helpful information.[4] With a knowledge of biomechanics and your specific foot type, you can make a better choice than shopping blindly.

A biomechanically efficient runner lands on the heel and rolls inward with a slight pronation to absorb shock. Over-pronation is the often excessive inward roll of the foot as you push off on the toe. Supination is the outward roll of the foot as you push off the toe.

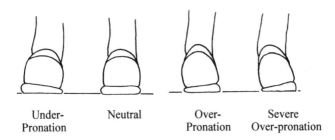

| Under-Pronation | Neutral | Over-Pronation | Severe Over-pronation |

Depending on whose advice you take when looking for shoes, you may do one of several things.

☞ Have a friend watch you run or even videotape your feet to determine how they land, how much you pronate, and your general form. This, with the wear patterns on your old shoes, can help determine whether you should look for shoes which compensate for under-pronation, over-pronation, severe over-pronation, or whether can get by with shoes for neutral pronators. Use this information to select shoes from one of four categories: flexibility trainers for under-pronators, neutral trainers for neutral pronators, stability trainers for over-pronators, and motion-control trainers for severe over-pronators.[5]

☞ First match your running and biomechanical needs, including your most common running surface into one of five categories: motion-control, stability, cushioned, lightweight training, or trails. Secondly, determine whether your foot type is normal, flat, or high-arched (found below). Use this information to select shoes from that category.[6]

Take your old shoes with you when you shop for new shoes. The wear patterns on the soles can help you, or the salesperson, determine how you run and the best shoes for your running style. Normal wear is on the outer heel and the across the ball of the foot. Pronators show wear on the outer heel and the inner forward side of the shoe. Supinators typically show wear on the heel to the forefoot along the outer edge of the shoe.

A key to getting a good fit in running shoes is understanding your foot type. To determine your foot type, walk on a hard surface with wet, bare feet to see your imprint. You should fit one of three arch types.

☞ Normal arched feet leave an imprint that shows the forefoot and heel connected, but with an inward curve at the arch. These runners will typically do best in a semicurved last shoe since they are generally efficient in their running gait and do not need motion-control shoes.

☞ Flat-arched feet leave an imprint which is almost complete without an inward curve at the arch. These runners will typically do best in a semicurved or straight last shoe which offers good stability and/or motion control. These runners are often over-pronators.

☞ High-arched feet leave an imprint which shows the forefoot and heel connected by a very narrow curve at the arch. These runners will typically do best in a curved last shoe with good cushioning. These runners are often supinators (under-pronators).

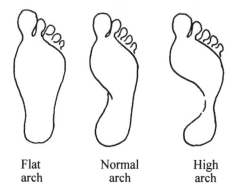

Flat   Normal   High
arch   arch   arch

Shop around until you find running shoes that feel right on your feet. A correct fit will help in blister prevention. Valerie Doyle remembers her fight to beat blisters. When she learned how to buy shoes that fit properly she found they solved her blister problem. The same applies to fitting boots. Studies have found that tight footwear can increase the forces exerted by the shoe or boot on the foot, which increases blister probability, while loose-fitting footwear increases the movement of the foot inside the shoe or boot, which causes increased friction forces on the foot, which in turn increases blister probability.[7]

You may find shoes that fit well with one exception. The toes may pinch or you may have corns or bunions that create pressure in specific areas. Some runners will cut slits into the side or the toe boxes of shoes to provide a better fit. Other runners will actually cut out a portion of the shoe over the problem area. If you do this, be careful not to sacrifice the integrity of the shoe. Be aware of the additional problem this may cause. Dirt and small rocks can easily get into the shoe and lead to hot spots and blisters.

If you have narrow or wide feet, consider shopping for shoes or boots which offer variable lacing capabilities. These shoes and boots will have lace eyelets which are not lined up in an up-and-down row but spaced horizontally farther apart. See the chapter *Lacing Options* on page 89 for information on how to lace for different types of feet.

When you shop for shoes or boots, run your fingers around the inside to determine whether there are any rough spots, overlapping or raised seams, or other potential pressure points that could cause hot spots or blisters. These may be able to be rubbed flat or softened. Ask the store for another pair to determine if the spots are common to that style or just one particular shoe or boot.

If you have difficulty finding quality shoes that fit your particular type of foot problems, consider searching for a certified pedorthist. A pedorthist is an individual trained to work on the fit or modification of shoes and orthotics to alleviate foot problems caused by disease, overuse, or injury. He or she may be able to modify your running shoe(s) or boot(s) for a better fit. Look in the telephone book or ask your orthopedist or podiatrist for references.

The American Academy of Orthopaedic Surgeons gives suggestions for buying shoes. Foremost, they remind us that shoes should always conform to the shape of your feet, your feet should never be forced to conform to the shape of a pair of shoes. Their suggestions apply equally well to buying boots. Suggestions include:

☞ Fit new shoes to your larger foot.
☞ Try on and fully lace both shoes.
☞ Judge a shoe by how it fits on your foot, not by the marked size.
☞ Try on shoes at the end of the day, preferably after running or walking, because your feet normally swell and become larger after standing and sitting during the day.
☞ Wear the same type of socks that you will wear for running or hiking.
☞ You should be able freely to wiggle all your toes.

☞ There should be a firm grip of the shoe to your heel.

☞ Make sure you do not feel the seams or stitching inside the shoes.

Long-distance hikers may find their feet enlarging by one or more sizes while on a long thru-hike. Ultrarunners can experience an enlargement in their feet of several sizes in a multi-day event. Remember to allow enough toe space when buying either shoes or boots. Allow about a 1/2" space between the end of the longest toe and the front of the shoe. When the foot is in the shoe, the arch naturally flattens. Since the heel is held in place by the heel of the shoe, the foot can only move forward. If the shoe does not have this bit of extra space in the toe box, the toes become cramped. Toenail problems, blisters, and calluses may develop. This important consideration is the fit problem most often overlooked.

Insoles

Insoles are designed to provide extra support and/or cushioning during running and hiking. Some models are molded to cradle the heel, support the arch, and cushion the forefoot while others have only an arch support, or are flat. Replacement insoles are to be used in place of your shoe's standard insole. Many replacement insoles offer better heel support, shock absorption, energy return, and reduction of friction than the insoles which come with the shoes. The insoles listed below are typically found in running, camping, and sporting goods stores. Ask to see their product catalogs if their shelf stock is low or if you are looking for a particular type.

If you have tried changing socks and other techniques to decrease your chance of blisters, try changing insoles. You may find that a particular brand or type of insole may be better at reducing blisters on your feet. This is usually due to the fabric or components of the insole. Insoles are not made to last forever. Check them for breakdown and replace them when necessary. This will depend on how you run and hike, and your mileage.

Replacement insoles are not sold as corrective footbeds. If a particular brand or style of insole is uncomfortable, try another type. These insoles are not meant to be used as orthotics. Always consult with an orthopedist or podiatrist if you are having recurring foot problems.

If you purchase insoles and they are too tight in certain areas of your feet, inquire with your local shoe repair shop or a pedorthist about thinning them with a belt sander.

Hapad Comf-Orthotic® Hapad makes full-length and 3/4-length insoles. The original contoured Comf-Orthotic full-length and 3/4-length insoles are made from Hapad featherweight wool. The coiled, spring-like wool fibers provide firm and resilient support while providing arch, metatarsal, and heel cushioning. The full-length contoured Comf-Orthotic Sports Replacement Insole is made in three layers with a moisture wicking suede top, a ventilated Poron® middle layer for shock absorption, and a bottom of Microcel® "Puff," a self-molding footbed. The insole includes a metatarsal bar to relieve pressure at the ball of the foot, a medial arch support to limit pronation, and a heel cup for stability and control of the foot and ankle. For more information contact Hapad, Inc.

Sof Sole® Sof Sole by IMPLUS is a line of replacement insoles made with the Implus® Cellular Cushioning System. This open-cell material provides superior shock absorption while allowing air and moisture to pass through. Additionally, these insoles contain a biocide additive to retard the growth of bacteria and fungus. Choose from Sof Runn Plus (a molded insole ideal for running), Sof Arch & Heel Support, Sof Heel Cup, or Sof Gel Pad or Sof Heel Pad for the heel.

Spenco® Spenco make several types of replacement insoles for runners. Choose from a molded full length cushioning system of Polysorb® for best shock absorption and energy return, a closed cell neoprene arch cushion in full- or 3/4-length, a slip-in flat insole, or a full-length gel cushion insole.

Spectrum Sports Inc. Spectrum Sports makes an assortment of replacement insoles. Choose from the Ultra Sole, Graphite Arch, Ultra Sole, Sorbo Lite and Sorboair made with Sorbothane® (a visco elastic polymer with high impact shock absorption), the Silver Liner model made from a lightweight polyurethane foam, the Summit Hiking and Backpacking insole with Sorbothane, or a neoprene 3/4-length arch support.

Superfeet   Superfeet footbeds are made in three systems: trim-to-fit, replacement-fit, and custom-fit. Their corrective shape and design offers a stabilizer cap which provides excellent support and stability to the bone structure of the foot, allowing the foot muscles to function more efficiently. In the trim-to-fit system, the low- and high-profile models are made for running and hiking. Replacement system footbeds are the lower end of the line without the stabilizer cap. For information on stores which have the custom-fit system, contact Superfeet.

Some boot companies like Merrell and Vasque also make insoles. Check your local store for these and other insoles.

Part Two

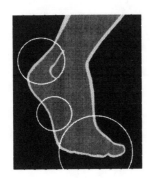

Preventative Maintenance

6

Making Preventative Maintenance Work

"The 6th Law Of Running Injuries:
Treat the Cause, Not the Effect.
Because each running injury has a cause, it follows that the injury
can never be cured until the causative factors are eliminated."
Tim Noakes, MD, *The Lore of Running.*[8]

How true — any running injury can only be cured *only* after the
cause is found and eliminated. All of us who run, hike, or adventure
race at some point have problems or injuries with our feet. This
section on preventative maintenance is lengthy because there are
many factors which can help prevent the cause of foot problems and
injuries.

Preventative maintenance is *proactive*. Time spent being
proactive in preventing problems will pay off in the long run. Taking
a *proactive* approach will mean less time being *reactive* to problems
when you often do not have the time to spare nor readily available
materials.

The key to making preventative maintenance work is to find
what works for you in the environment where you will use it. In
other words, try the fix where it will be used. When you are trying to
find what works for you on trails, running on roads will not typically
provide the same results as actually running on trails. I made my
own gaiters for trail running after determining that the dirt getting
into my shoes was causing hot spots and blisters. I never would have

made that determination without running on trails. Likewise, walking around town while wearing a backpack and your hiking boots is never the same as hiking on a rocky trail with uneven terrain. That may help to break in the boots but will not give the same feeling as a rough rocky trail.

Your feet will respond to training in the same way your legs respond. Increasing your running or hiking time by increments will allow your feet time to adapt to the added stresses of the additional mileage. Suddenly doubling your mileage will likely lead to potential problems. If you are working up to a marathon, an ultra, longer ultras, or a multi-day hike, do back-to-back training days to work your feet into their best possible condition.

7

The Components of Preventative Maintenance

The one problem with our feet we most often experience, that drives us crazy, and costs us time and, in some cases, unfulfilled dreams — is blisters. These chapters on preventative maintenance deal with keeping our feet healthy by preventing the "dreaded" blisters.

Preventative maintenance works through a combination of components. Socks, powders, lubricants, skin tougheners, taping, orthotics, nutrition for the feet, proper hydration, anti-perspirants for the feet, gaiters, laces, and frequent sock and shoe changes are among the preventative components available to fix foot problems.

Imagine a triangle with heat, friction, and moisture at its three sides. These three factors combine to make the skin more susceptible to blisters. Heat and moisture, in the presence of friction, lead to blisters.

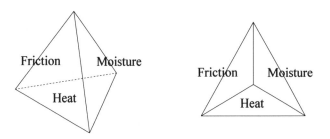

The three factors of blister formation

Dr. David Hannaford, a podiatrist and runner, stresses that "If you eliminate any one of the three factors, you eliminate the blister." The triangle with these three factors, heat, friction, and moisture, sits on a base which has two levels.

Each level of the base is a circle made up of components which can prevent these three factors from forming. Closest to the triangle is the top circle with the components of socks, powders, and lubricants — the first line of defense against blisters. Friction, which produces heat, can be reduced by wearing a sock with wicking properties, either alone or with an outer sock, or by using powders or lubricant. Moisture can be reduced with the wicking properties of certain socks and by using powders to keep the feet dry.

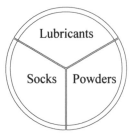

The top inner circle of blister prevention components

Socks are either single- or double-layer construction. Some single-layer socks, particularly those without wicking properties, allow friction to develop between the feet and the socks, which in turn can create blisters. Double-layer socks allow the sock layers to move against each other, which reduces friction between the feet and the first sock layer.

Powders reduce friction by reducing moisture on the skin which in turn reduces friction between the feet and the socks.

Lubricants create a shield, either greasy or non-greasy, to areas of the skin which are in contact during motion. This lubricant shield reduces chafing, which in turn reduces friction.

The bottom of the base is an outer circle made up of components that play a strong supporting role in preventative maintenance. This outer circle is made up of components including skin tougheners, taping, orthotics, nutrition for the feet and proper hydration, anti-perspirants for the feet, gaiters, laces, and frequent sock and shoe changes. Each can contribute to the prevention of blisters and other problems. You could argue that these outer components should be identified as major components, and to some extent you may be right. Some components may be more important for your feet than for mine. The trick is to determine what we each need to keep our feet healthy under the stresses of our particular sport.

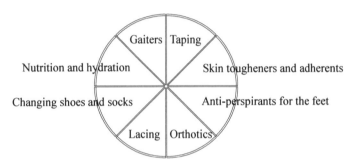

The bottom outer circle of blister prevention components

Skin tougheners form a coating to protect and toughen the skin. These products also help tape and blister patches adhere better to the skin.

Taping provides a barrier between the skin and socks so friction is reduced. Proper taping adds an extra layer of skin (the tape) to the foot to prevent hot spots and blisters. Taping can also be a treatment if hot spots and blisters do develop.

Orthotics help maintain the foot in a functionally neutral position so arch and pressure problems are relieved. Small pads for the feet may also help correct foot imbalances and pressure points. Nutrition for the feet includes creams and lotions so dry and callused feet are softened. The result is softer and smoother skin.

Proper hydration can help reduce swelling of the feet so the occurrence of hot spots and blisters is reduced.

Anti-perspirants for the feet helps those with sweaty feet by reducing the moisture that makes the feet more prone to blisters.

Gaiters provide protection against dirt, rocks, and grit. These irritants cause friction and blisters as shoes and socks become dirty.

Shoe and boot laces often cause friction or pressure problems. Adjusting laces can relieve this friction and pressure and make footwear more comfortable.

Frequent sock changes help keep the feet in good condition. Wet or moist socks can cause problems. Changing the socks also gives opportunity to reapply either powder or lubricant and deal with any hot spots before they become blisters. Sometimes shoes are also changed as they become overly dirty or wet.

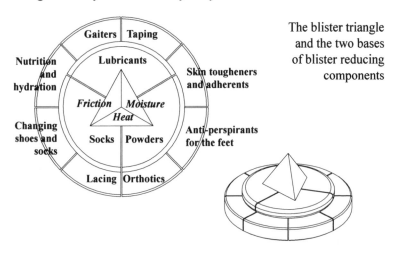

The blister triangle and the two bases of blister reducing components

Each runner and hiker needs to find what combination works for them. One may use Vaseline, another may use Zeasorb powder, while another may pre-tape his feet. They each may use one of many types and styles of socks. Ultrarunner Dave Scott claims his feet are often "... as soft as a baby's bottom" after the 100 mile Western States Endurance Run. Dave has found that he rarely gets foot problems. He trims his toenails, uses a small amount of Vaseline, and regularly changes his shoes and socks. That is what works for him. At the other extreme is the runner who has the skin falling off his feet from midsoles to heels. One hiker may end a six day hike having had a few simple foot problems while another may have suffered with major problems the whole trip. Determine what foot problems you normally experience, study this book, and then begin the task of finding what works best for your feet.

Ultrarunner Tim Twietmeyer has won the grueling 100 mile Western States Endurance Run four times while accumulating 15 silver belt buckles for sub-24 hour finishes. Over the past five years, in addition to running ultras, he has enjoyed fastpacking in the California High Sierras. He has found the differences interesting.

A week before running a 100-mile trail ultra Tim trims his toenails as short as possible. The morning of the run he coats his feet with lanolin to reduce friction, provide warmth if running in snow or through water, and make his skin more resilient to getting all wrinkled. Then he pulls on a pair of Thorlo Ultrathin socks. His strategy is "... that the more sock you wear, the more moisture close to the foot. The more moisture the more blisters and skin problems." He usually wears the same pair of shoes and socks the entire way. Tim acknowledges "... my feet don't usually have problems, and when they do, I'm close enough to the end to gut it out."

Tim has found that fastpacking affects his feet differently. When he did the John Muir Trail in 1992 (five days and ten hours to do 210 miles), his feet were trashed more than ever before. His group of five experienced ultrarunners averaged 14 hours per day on the rough trail. Tim remembers, "We covered the ground so fast that my feet swelled and I almost couldn't get my shoes on the last day." He used the same strategy of lanolin and thin socks. Instead of running shoes he chose lightweight hiking boots. Foot repair became the group's daily ritual as the 40 mile days took their toll. They realized that "... an important strategy for keeping our feet from getting any worse was to get that first piece of duct tape on in just the right spot and making it stick. If we did that, our feet held up pretty well." By the end of the fifth day the last piece of duct tape had been used on their feet. Tim's cardinal rule for fastpacking is to "Keep your feet dry." While that can be hard to do when fighting afternoon thunderstorms, if your feet are wet too long, it's only a matter of time before they blister. Whether running ultras or fastpacking, Tim knows the importance of keeping his feet healthy and has experimented to find what works well for his feet.

We need to understand the importance of other elements which contribute to preventative maintenance. These elements are discussed in *Part Three: Treatments* of this book. Proper strength training and conditioning will help make the foot and ankle stronger and more resistant to sprains and strains. Good care of the skin will help prevent calluses. Quality insoles and orthotics can help prevent or relieve the problems of plantar fasciitis, Achilles tendinitis, heel pain, metatarsalgia, Morton's neuroma, Morton's foot, sesamoiditis, corns, and bunions. Good-fitting footwear will help prevent problems with toenails, arches, and blisters. In short, everything you put on or around your foot becomes related to how well your foot functions.

8

Socks

Socks perform four basic functions: cushioning, protection, warmth, and absorbing moisture off the skin. The sock fabric and weave will determine how well they do in each of the four areas. Socks made from synthetic fabrics wick moisture away from the skin and through the sock to its outer surface where it can evaporate.

Some athletes wear the common cotton crew sock while others swear by synthetic socks or synthetic double layer socks. Each method has its reasons. If cotton crew socks work for you, continue using them. If however, you are plagued by hot spots and/or blisters, consider trying other types of socks. Cotton tube socks should always be avoided for both running and hiking because of their loose fit.

For my first 24-hour track run I wore thick cotton socks and used gobs of Vaseline on my feet. That was what everyone else seemed to be doing, so that was what I did. It didn't take long for blisters to develop on my heels and toes which reduced me to a slow walk. Even so, I managed to get in a respectable 103 miles. Without the early foot problems, I am sure I could have done another ten miles. I learned the hard way what did not work on my feet and set out to find what did work.

Clean socks can feel heavenly. When hiking, wash yesterday's socks and let them dry on the back of your pack. Try to change socks several times during a 100-mile run and once during a

50-mile run. During multi-day events, try to change socks several times a day. If clean socks are unavailable from your crew, try to wash the dirty socks so they are clean for later use.

Types of Socks

Socks come in a variety of fabrics: cotton, cotton blends, synthetics, silk, wool and wool blends, and fleece. An overview of these materials provides insights into their uses. Read the product information on the sock's packaging and try several types to find those that work best for you.

☞ **Cotton** — A 100% cotton sock provides no wicking or insulating properties and therefore moisture is retained against the skin. In damp or wet cotton, your feet are generally wet, cold, and more prone to blistering.

☞ **Cotton blends** — A cotton blend, with cotton as the main product, offers a limited advantage over a pure cotton sock. Cotton may be blended with Lycra®, nylon, rayon, and acrylic.

☞ **Fleece** — Fleece socks are soft, provide exceptional warmth, and dry faster than wool.

☞ **Synthetics** — The newer synthetic material socks offer protection against blisters caused by moisture, poor fit, hot spots, slippage, or friction. These are made of hydrophobic materials which means they don't like moisture or water. Moisture-wicking fabrics like Capilene®, Coolmax®, Olefin, or polypropylene wick moisture and perspiration away from the skin to the outer layer of the sock. Synthetic insulators like Hollofil®, Thermax®, or Thermastat™ help provide insulation. Some of these socks are single layer while others are double layer. Most of the socks use one of the above fabrics blended with cotton, nylon, Lycra spandex, or acrylic.

☞ **Silk** — Silk socks are slick and generally used as liners. With low wicking properties and low heat retention they do not dry as fast as the newer synthetics.

☞ **Wool** — Wool wicks while retaining its cushioning but can be scratchy and rough.

☞ **Wool blends** — Wool blends make for a more comfortable fit and a tougher-wearing sock. Socks made from worsted wool are soft and durable. Merino wool, from sheep with a lighter and softer coat, is less resilient but very soft and comfortable. Wool may also be blended with other fabrics.

The weave of the sock will vary depending on the material. Socks will range from a loose weave to a dense weave. The loose weave will feel coarse and provide less insulation. The dense weave will feel softer and generally offers more cushioning. Put your hand inside a sock and stretch the foot portion with your fingers to see the weave. Denser-weave socks will show little space between the fibers.

Double-layer socks are used to help reduce or eliminate the likelihood of blisters developing. The two layers moving against each other instead of against the skin reduces skin friction. Most double-layer socks utilize wicking properties to move moisture away from the feet. Before wearing any double-layer sock, align the layers with your hand and then roll the socks on the foot for the best fit.

Buy socks that fit your feet. The heels, toes, and length should fit snugly without sagging or being stretched too tight. Socks that are too big will bunch up and cause friction and skin irritation. Socks that are too small can cause the toes and joints to rub harder against the socks. Turn them inside out and look at the toe seams. Avoid those with bulky seams because they can rub, causing hot spots and blisters. After buying socks be sure to try them on with your shoes or boots to be sure they fit together and are not too tight. Remember also to discard socks when they become threadbare and too thin to provide their advertised benefits.

Many stores offer a basket of socks to use when trying on shoes and boots. Try to avoid these and instead use your own socks when shopping. This way you get to feel the fit with your personal socks and avoid picking up a foot fungus from another shopper.

The following sections identify specific *Running Socks*, *Hiking Socks*, *Sock Liners*, *High-Technology Socks*, and *Sandal Socks*. Review each of these sections for an overview of the wide range of available socks. Many of the socks may be used for running, hiking, and adventure racing. Check them out at a store near you to feel them and read their packaging information.

Running Socks

The following are a sampling of running socks typically available in running stores. Check your local store for the types they carry. If the store does not stock the types described here, or that you have seen in a magazine, ask the staff if they can order other types.

BaySix BaySix offers either single- or double-layer socks in ankle and crew lengths. Their Wonderspun™ yarns made from rayon wrapped in nylon provide wicking properties that transfer heat and moisture away from the foot. The double-layer sock is designed to allow the layers to move against each other, reducing the friction against the skin.

Fox River Fox River makes a Coolmax triathlon sock.

Ridgeview® Ridgeview offers crew and ankle-high socks of a Coolmax, stretch nylon, and elastic combination.

Runique™ AA-R Hosiery makes the original double-layer sock from Wonderspun® yarns with stretch nylon and spandex.

Thorlo® Thorlo uses their Thorlo System Fit™ to make socks for specific sports activities. The combination of acrylic and stretch nylon helps to reduce blisters and other foot discomforts. The socks have a combination of resilient, spongy pads at the ball and heel and a lower-density pad at the arch for a contour fit and reduction in bulk. The socks use Foot Health™ yarns to wick moisture away from the foot. Choose between highly cushioned or thinner, lightweight socks.

Wigwam® Wigwam offers a complete line of socks for specific sports activities: running, triathlons, cycling, etc. Their Ultimax® sock line uses Olefin, a moisture-absorbing acrylic, nylon, and Lycra spandex. Another style uses a combination of Coolmax, cotton, and stretch nylon.

Wrightsock™ Wrightsock offers a double-layer sock made of nylon and Coolmax. The two layers move against each other to reduce the friction against the skin.

Other Sock Options Other types of sock and combinations of socks that have been tried include:

☞ Will Uher likes rock climber's socks that are thin and fit snugly on his feet.

☞ Any two pairs of socks can be used together, as an inner and outer layer. Usually, the thinner layer is worn inside.

☞ Ankle-high nylons. Yes, nylons — as an inner sock! Sid Snyder found that by wearing ankle high nylons under his Thorlo socks he does not get blisters. No tape and no Vaseline — just the nylons. He had blistered so bad on another long trail event that he was on crutches for three days and knew he had to try something new. Be sure to try this combination before a competitive event. Try them with the sock you normally wear, preferably a wicking sock. When using nylons for trail running or hiking, be sure to try them on uphills and downhills since some individuals may be bothered by the slippery smooth nylon.

☞ Camping stores carry socks that can be used for running. New socks are continually being designed. Acorn makes a fleece Tekna-Sport sock with excellent moisture management. Dahlgren offers a Dri-Stride Trail Fitness sock with moisture management zones. Smartwool makes a Ultra Thin soft merino wool and nylon moisture wicking sock.

Hiking Socks

Hiking socks are different from running socks. Hikers most often wear crew or high-top socks. Some wear a wool outer sock with a liner that has wicking properties. Hikers could also try the thinner double-layer wicking socks in a crew top style. These wear well, wick moisture away, and are made to reduce the possibility of blisters.

Pacific Crest Trail hiker Matthew Jankowicz used to get blisters, especially on long hikes over 20 miles a day. He tried tape, moleskin, and different kinds of boots. Finally, he switched to wearing three pair of socks and it worked. He uses one pair of wicking socks over which he wears two pair of boot socks. Matthew says, "I know some people think I'm crazy but it works very well for me and I have hiked thousands of miles this way without getting any blisters on my feet."

The following list of sock companies is provided to show how diverse the field is and how many different types of socks there are to choose from. There are also many more companies not listed. Each company introduces new versions of their socks each year. New fabrics and combinations of fabrics make the sock selection ever changing. Your camping and backpacking store will have displays of many of these socks. Investigate your socks options and talk to others about their preferences to determine which socks may be best for your hiking needs.

Acorn Fleece Socks   Acorn Products make fleece socks which can be used for hiking. Made with Polartec® fleece fabric these socks provide lightweight warmth and rapid drying. Sock options include an Outdoor Versa-Tek™, the Versa-Tek 200 2-way stretch socks or the Tekna-Sport.

Bridgedale   Fabric combinations may include Coolmax, cotton, nylon, wool, or Lycra spandex. Sock options include the Advanced Technical Leisure, Explorer Boot Length, Coolmax Hiking, and Advanced Technical Walking Boot Length.

Dahlgren   Dahlgren Footwear makes Dri-Stride socks with their Climate Knit™ system. The socks have Patented Zones™ of wool, cotton, and Dursaspun™ Smart Yarns® to control temperature and provide wicking of moisture. Sock options include Hiking, Light Hiking, and Trail Fitness styles.

Fox River   Fox River socks are made with their Wick Dry® system. Individual sock fabrics include combinations of acrylic, Coolmax, stretch nylon, worsted wool, cotton, or polypropylene. Sock options include hiking socks: the Meridian, Endro, and the Tramper; and trekking socks: Sierra and the Explorer.

Patagonia   Patagonia offers socks with their soft, quick drying, and moisture wicking Capilene. Fabric combinations include Capilene, worsted wool, and stretch nylon. Sock options include Lightweight, Mid-Weight, and Expedition Weight Capilene.

REI Socks   REI makes a complete line of socks with their label. Individual sock fabrics include combinations of acrylic, stretch nylon, worsted wool, cotton, Lycra spandex, or polypropylene. Sock options include Long Rugged Ragg, Rugged Terrain, Cotton Wool Ragg, Canyon, Classic Ragg, Outdoor, and Wool Backpacker.

Smartwool™   Smartwool socks from Duke Designs are made from very soft Merino wool and Lycra and use their Active-Fit™ system. Sock options include an Expedition Trekking, Hiking, and Sport Trek.

Thorlo   Thorlo uses their Thorlo System Fit to make socks for specific sports activities. The socks are made from a combination of fabrics and each may include acrylic, Coolmax, stretch nylon, Lycra spandex, or wool. Sock options include the Extreme Weather Over-the-Calf, Light Hiking Crew, Hiking Crew, Light Trekking Crew, Trekking Crew, and Coolmax Hiker.

Wigwam   Wigwam offers a complete line of socks for hiking, many with their Wonder-Wick™ Foot Drying System. Individual sock fabrics include combinations of acrylic, Olefin, Hollofil polyester, Coolmax, stretch nylon, wool, cotton, polypropylene, or Lycra. Sock options include Ultimax Hiking and Outdoor, Ultimax Rugged Outdoor, Mid-Weight Backpacking, Outdoor Heavyweight Wool Ragg, Canada Boot, Norway Ragg, Wander, All-Terrain Coolmax Crew, and the Merino Wool Light Hiker.

Sock Liners

Sock liners are thin, smooth, and are made to be worn under a heavier insulating or cushioning sock, typically wool. Liners should wick moisture away from the foot and into the outer sock. A liner will perform with the outer sock the same as the double layer socks. Friction will occur between the two layers and not against the skin, reducing the chance of blisters. When shopping for liners, look for a style with wicking properties. While many runners are converting to the double-layer socks, some still prefer a two-sock system using liners.

Fox River   The Fox River Wick & Dry Sockliner is made from polypropylene.

Helly-Hansen Polypro Liners   These polypropylene liners are available in several thicknesses which offer options in use with outer socks.

Patagonia Capilene Liners   P a t a g o n i a ' s
Capilene Crew Liner socks are durable, thin, and fast-drying. These
are made from Capilene polyester and stretch nylon.

Wigwam   Wigwam offers several sock liners. The
Liner Sock is made with the Thermastat Wonder-Wick Foot Dry
System to protect feet against cold and blisters. They also offer a
Coolmax Liner and an Ultimax Liner for Outdoor and Ski with a
moisture control system. The Gobi Plus and Gobi Polypro liners are
made from polypropylene. The Stretch Mojave® Liner is made from
worsted wool, stretch nylon, and Lycra spandex while the Stretch
Solaris® Liner is made from pure Chinese Silk and nylon.

Z-Dry One®   Z Knit makes a Z-Dry One inner
sock made from polypropylene and nylon.

High-Technology Oversocks

Oversocks are special high-technology socks that combine waterproof technology and the comfort of traditional socks into a somewhat baggy-looking sock. They were developed for anyone who
participates in outdoor activities where the feet are exposed to
water. Widely used by hunters and fishermen, they are being discovered by runners, hikers, and adventure racers. Feet are kept dry and
comfortable even though the shoes or boots may be soaked and
muddy.

National champion ultrarunner Roy Pirrung tested the high-
technology oversock SealSkinz® for a year in all kinds of weather.
Roy recalls his win at the 100 KM Glacial Trail Run, a grueling race
through the wet Kettle Moraine State Forest in Wisconsin. "It had
rained the day before and conditions were sloppy. As other runners
stopped every 10 miles to change their wet socks, I just raced ahead.
I ended up finishing the race within 25 seconds of the course record,
and without any blisters." In wet and cold conditions, oversocks can
work wonders. Roy found that SealSkinz have helped him to train
outside in minus 25-degree weather with a wind-chill factor of minus 80. His feet "... stayed warm, dry and comfortable."

Oversocks work best when used with a Coolmax or other wicking material sock liner. This further enhances moisture dispersion as well as comfort. Care must be taken when pulling the socks on or off to avoid tearing the inner membrane. A torn membrane will allow water to penetrate at the tear site.

Ideally, oversocks should not be submersed in water over the cuffs. Once water has gone down the leg into the sock, the wicking process slows or stops, depending on the amount of water in the sock. Over time, the body's heat combined with the wicking action of the Coolmax liner may dry the inside of the socks, but this depends on both the amount of water inside the sock and the degree of activity. Roy recommends wearing tights over the cuffs to provide a covering seal.

REI/Gore-Tex® Oversocks   The REI/Gore-Tex Oversocks are waterproof, breathable and designed to be worn over a pair of thin wicking socks. The socks have a Gore-Tex® membrane laminated between inner and outer fabric layers. The inner seams are sealed with Gore Seam™ tape. The sole and back panel are made of a non-stretch Gore-Tex® fabric to increase durability and prevent slippage. The upper panels are stretchable Gore-Tex fabric for flexibility and conformity to the foot's shape. A spandex cuff helps the socks stay up. When wearing these socks, watch for skin irritations caused by the inner seams. These socks are available through all REI stores or through REI mail order.

SealSkinz® Waterproof MVT Socks   SealSkinz socks from Dupont® are seamless waterproof socks that use moisture vapor transpiration (MVT) technology. The socks are made in a thin, lightweight, three-layer design. An inner Coolmax or Thermastat liner wicks moisture away from the skin while a middle layer of vapor-permeable membrane allows perspiration to escape and prevents water from entering. The outer layer uses nylon for abrasion resistance and durability. The Lycra spandex cuff ensures the socks will stay up. Their seamless design gives them a positive edge in preventing blisters.

The All-Season Socks are made for general wear and use Coolmax as a wicking liner. The Insulated Socks are made for cold conditions to protect feet from extreme temperatures and use

Thermastat as a liner to both wick away moisture and retain body heat. An Over-the-Calf sock is also available. An All-Sport version in ankle and crew lengths is perfect for runners. The socks are made in small, medium, large and extra large. SealSkinz can be ordered through sporting good stores and outdoor specialty stores. Contact Dupont for the dealer nearest you.

Many of the Eco-Challenge Adventure Race teams use SealSkinz socks to keep their feet free of blisters, abrasions caused by dirt and grime, and the effects of water immersion during their long, multi-day competition.

Seirus Neo-Sock® and StormSock™   The Seirus Neo-Sock provides warmth from closed-cell insulation for winter activities. It is made from four-way stretch neoprene with breathable macro porous technology to prevent moisture buildup while sealing in body heat. These socks have a nylon fabric on either side of the neoprene which allows moisture to pass through. The StormSock has an outer layer of Lycra, an inner membrane of high-technology Weather Shield™ that stops wind and water, and is lined with Polartec fleece. Both socks have seams which should be checked for waterproofing. These socks are made by Seirus Innovative Accessories.

Sandal Socks

The advent of newer and better designs of sport sandals make them popular for general wear. Some of the better styles can be used for running or hiking. Multi-day hikers can wear sandals in camp as a refreshing change from their heavier hiking boots. While regular socks can be worn with sandals, specific sandal socks are offered.

Acorn Fleece Socks   Acorn Products make a Polartec Sandal Sock of fleece for lightweight warmth and rapid drying.

Bridgedale   Bridgedale makes two socks for sandals. The ankle length Advanced Technical Sandal sock is made of Coolmax, combed cotton, nylon, and Lycra. The Dingle sock is made from combed cotton, nylon, and Lycra.

The Option of Not Wearing Socks

In 1973 a running magazine advertised "New, lean, and luxurious — the first sockless athletic shoe." After three years of development, Bare Foot Gear, offered the "Original Sockless Shoe" with prime leather inside and out, no staples or nails, no seams or ridges, and no textiles to touch your foot. Just unpainted and unsealed leather. Cupping the foot only at the heel and instep, it offered a large space up front for flexion and good air circulation. With a drier foot, it advertised, friction is minimized. Looking at the ad today, we might find humor in the ad's statement "Most men prefer no socks because of the sheer maleness of the feel." I never saw the shoe.

There is the option, like the shoe designers hoped people would buy into, of not wearing socks. Some prefer this option. Matt Mahoney found the best way to prevent blisters was to train for them. Walking barefoot and sometimes running barefoot on grass, dirt, or sand toughened the skin on his feet. He does not wear socks with shoes, but rotates between several brands of shoes to develop calluses at every spot that could rub. Matt found that socks caused his feet to slide around inside his shoes and he couldn't grip the trail on steep hills. When he finds spots rubbing, he uses tape, Vaseline, or Compeed.

This type of barefoot running or running in shoes without socks takes time and careful monitoring of your feet to avoid problems. Matt has conditioned his feet by walking a mile barefoot on roads every day. He estimates he runs 15% of the time barefoot on grass and dirt and the other 85% in shoes without socks. He has strengthened the small muscles and tendons in his feet. The skin on the bottom of his feet has toughened to provide some degree of protection for running barefoot. Gradually toughen your feet with short periods of barefoot walking before trying to run barefoot. If trying to go without socks, check your shoes for rough seams or ridges which can cut into your feet. Like Matt, use tape or a lubricant on areas that rub. Matt strongly believes we need to, "Learn to run in simple shoes, sandals, or barefoot as people have done for thousands of years before Nike."

Walking and running barefoot can be an excellent way to condition your feet in order to prevent blisters when you do wear boots or shoes.

9

Powders

There are powders and then there are powders. Corn starch and talcum powder have been used for years as foot powders, but times and powders have changed. Having tried a super absorbent powder, I would never again use a plain powder. Powders can be effective in reducing moisture on the feet. Their effectiveness depends on their ability to absorb moisture while not caking into clumps. Clumps can cause skin irritations and blisters. When using powders, remember to reapply the powder at regular intervals or after the feet have been exposed to water. If you have problems with athlete's foot or other skin problems, use a medicated powder.

Gold Bond®   Gold Bond is a medicated body powder which contains active ingredients zinc oxide as a skin protector and menthol to cool and relieve itching. Use the extra-strength powder for maximum benefits in absorbing excessive moisture. Gold Bond is made by Chattem, Inc. and is available through your local drug store and pharmacy.

Bromi-Talc™   Gordon Laboratories makes Bromi-Talc, a triple action foot powder. Bromi-Talc contains potassium alum, an astringent that retards perspiration; bentonite, a highly absorbent agent; and the highest grade talc powder for absorption. Bromi-Talc Plus™ powder contains additional properties to control excessive foot odor. Available only by special order through your local drug store, pharmacy, or podiatrist from Gordon Laboratories.

Zeasorb®   The success of Zeasorb is in its super absorbent powder, which absorbs almost four times more moisture than plain talcum powder. Zeasorb contains talc, a highly absorbent polymer-carbohydrate acrylic copolymer, and microporous cellulose for super absorbency. This powder is very efficient and works without caking. The talc provides softness and lubrication to reduce friction and heat buildup. Their second powder, ZeasorbAF®, with miconazole nitrate 2%, provides broad antifungal therapy and moisture control. Look for it at drug stores or order it through your local pharmacy. For more information contact Stiefel Laboratories, Inc.

10

Lubricants

Like powders, there are lubricants and then there are lubricants. Two of the old time tried-and-true lubricants are Lanolin and Vaseline. However technology has led to new formulas. Many runners have discovered Bag Balm. Others make their own special formulas.

Robert Boeder used Andrew Lovy's formula on his feet in 1994 when he completed the Grand Slam of trail ultrarunning, running four 100-mile runs in 14 weeks. Robert comments that, "The idea is that these lotional charms will have the desired magical effect and blisters will not arise from my feet during the race."[9] This formula worked well for him. Since that time he switched to Bag Balm and then back to Vaseline, mainly because of its availability.

Studies have shown that lubricants may initially reduce friction but over long periods of time they may actually increase friction. After one hour the friction levels returned to their baseline factor and after three hours the friction levels were 35% above the baseline. As the lubricants are absorbed into the skin and into the socks, friction returns and increases.[10] What we must learn from this is the need to reapply lubricants at frequent intervals.

Use lubricants on your feet, hands, underarms, inner thighs, and nipples — anywhere you chafe. The important thing to remember about lubricants is to clean the old off before applying a new coating. This is especially true during trail runs and hiking when dust and dirt buildup can foul the lubricant with grit. Wipe off the old stuff with a cleansing towelette or an alcohol wipe.

As always, try any new product before using it in a competitive event or taking it on a long hike. It is fool-hardy to buy something and count on it in competition or on a six-day hike without trying it first. It may not work for you. Try any lubricant on a small patch of skin to be sure you are not allergic to the ingredients.

Andrew Lovy's Formula   Andrew Lovy, in an article "New Blister Formula Revealed! Free!,"[11] shared a formula which he developed over several years. It has helped him solve his blister and friction problems. Take A and D Ointment, Vaseline, and Desitin ointment and mix together equal amounts. To this add Vitamin E cream and Aloe Vera cream (the thickness can be varied by the amount of these two ingredients). The result is a salve. For a thinner mixture, use Vitamin E and Aloe Vera ointment instead of the creams. Andrew recommends that the evening before your run, apply a thin layer to clean skin where friction occurs. In the morning, before you run, apply a more generous amount to friction areas. Add more to problem areas as necessary during the run. Shop around to find the ingredients in sizes appropriate for the total amount you want to mix.

Avon Silicone Glove   Avon makes this silicone cream for hands but it works equally well on feet. Its non-greasy and non-sticky formula lubricates while protecting against dryness and irritants as it softens. It is available in a handy 1.5 ounce tube. Contact your Avon sales representative for ordering information.

Bag Balm   Bag Balm, or what some runners call "udder balm," comes in a green tin which has become familiar to many runners. While Bag Balm is made and advertised for use on cow udders, it has found acceptance in sports circles. Consisting of a combination of lanolin, petrolatum, 8-hydroxy, and quinoline sulfate, many have found the salve to offer healing properties. It can be used on cracked, callused, or sore skin, or simply as a lubricant for your feet or other body areas. Available in one- or 10-ounce tins, it is usually found in feed stores and tack shops, but is becoming easier to find in many drug stores and hardware stores. For more information contact the Dairy Association Co. (east of the Rockies) or Smith Sales Service (west of the Rockies).

BodyGlide™   BodyGlide is a petroleum-free lubricant which protects against friction and skin irritation. This product comes in a "glide-on" applicator similar to a deodorant stick. BodyGlide is hypo-allergenic, waterproof, non-sticky, non-greasy so it will not clog pores, and long-lasting. Its main ingredients are triglycerides, aloe, and Vitamin E. Its applicator makes it awkward to use on toes but easy to apply to other areas. For more information contact BodyGlide.

Hydropel   Hydropel Protective Silicone Ointment is an excellent foot lubricant. It is made with 30% silicone, petrolatum, dimethicone, and aluminum starch octonylsuccinate. It is also rated effective as a protectant against poison ivy. Offered in a two-ounce or one-pound size. Available only by mail order through C & M Pharmacal. C & M distributes the same product to medical specialists under the name Protective Barrier Ointment in their Essential Care product line. For more information contact C & M.

Lanolin Cream   Some runners use lanolin cream on their feet. Lanolin hydrous is a natural topical skin emollient which lubricates, protects, and soothes. It usually comes in a small tube and may be found in most drug stores or pharmacies.

Runner's Lube™   Mueller makes Runner's Lube in a push-up tube. This anti-friction ointment contains lanolin, pain-relieving benzocaine, and zinc oxide. It can be found in sporting good stores. For more information contact Mueller Sports Medicine, Inc.

Skin-Lube®   Skin-Lube is a lubricating ointment which comes in a handy .55-ounce stick, a 2.75-ounce tube, or a one-pound jar. Its higher melting point gives it longer-lasting protection against blisters and chafing than petroleum jelly. Its main ingredients are petrolatum, zinc stearate, and silicone. Colorless and non-staining, it can be used on any friction-prone area of the body. It can be found in sporting good stores. For more information contact Cramer Products, Inc.

Sport Slick   Created by a sports physician, Sport Slick is a multi-purpose lubricant made for athletes. The gel is easily applied to the toes, feet, inner thighs, underarms, nipples, and lips. Sport Slick prevents blisters and chafing with antifriction polymers, silicone, and petrolatum which creates a silky feel. It also enriches the skin with Vitamin E and C, and sunscreen and contains the antifungal agent Tolnaftate 1%. Available in one-ounce packets and a four-ounce tube. For more information contact Sport Slick Products.

Sportsloob™   Sportsloob is a cream which protects the skin against chafing. Its main ingredients are liquid paraffin, white petroleum jelly, and emulsifying wax. The odorless and colorless cream is activated by body heat and perspiration, providing a non-greasy shield for areas of the skin that make contact during motion. It is advertised as effective for 12 to 18 hours. Available in a one-ounce tube. For more information contact Sportsloob.

Un-Petroleum® Jelly   For those wanting a lubricant without petroleum, try Un-Petroleum Jelly. Made from natural plant oils and waxes, its ingredients are castor oil, coconut oil, PG-3 beeswax, sorbitan tritearate, silica, tocopherol (Vitamin E), and natural flavors. It soothes and moisturizes dry skin, prevents chafing and windburn, and is a general purpose lubricant. Made by Autumn Harp, it is usually found in drug stores and health food stores.

Vaseline®   Vaseline is available in three formulas. The old-time standard is 100% pure petroleum jelly. Newer formulas include Creamy Vaseline® with Vitamin E and an anti-bacterial Medicated Vaseline®. The medicated formula, in particular, should be helpful for runner's feet, underarms, inner thighs, and nipples. Vaseline is available in most drug stores.

11

Skin Tougheners and Tape Adherents

Some athletes have found benefits against blisters by toughening the skin of their feet. Begin by spending time walking barefoot on various surfaces. Sandals, worn without socks, can build calluses, but be careful that the calluses do not become too thick or rough. As the skin is irritated, through exposure to rough surfaces, it thickens and calluses develop. Remember to keep calluses and roughened skin surfaces smooth by using creams, a pumice stone, or a foot file (see the chapters *Nutrition for the Feet* on page 79 and *Corns, Calluses, and Bunions* on page 145).

There are several products which can be used as skin tougheners or choose the tea and Betadine® soak. Several of the products can also be used as tape adherents to help your choice of tape or moleskin better adhere to the feet. Let the spray dry completely before applying any tape. Be sure to apply a light coating of powder over any dried sprayed area to counteract the adhesive. Without the adherent, most tapes and blister products will begin to peel off after an hour or two.

When using tincture of benzoin or a benzoin-based product, be sure to allow it time to dry. Generally three minutes' drying time is sufficient before applying any tape or blister product. Wet benzoin is very sticky and slippery. Tape and blister care products can move around on the foot and fold over on themselves creating problems. Socks can become glued to your feet and toes can stick together if you do not allow the benzoin time to dry.

Cramer Tuf-Skin®   Cramer's Tuf-Skin spray has been used for years by athletic trainers as a taping base. It is ideal for pre-taping and skin toughening. Its main ingredients are isopropyl alcohol, isobutane, resin, and benzoin. The original spray is available in an eight-ounce size while the colorless formula is available in four-, six-, and ten-ounces sizes. For more information contact Cramer Products, Inc.

Mueller Tuffner™ Clear Spray   This clear spray is used as a base for athletic taping, but is also identified as a skin toughener. Its main ingredients are acetone, 1,1,1-trichloroethanem isopropanol, resin, and tincture of benzoin. Look for this product at sporting good stores. For more information contact Mueller Sports Medicine, Inc.

New-Skin®   New-Skin Liquid Bandage is an antiseptic spray and antiseptic liquid that is useful as a skin protectant or toughener to prevent hot spots and blisters. It dries rapidly to form a tough protective cover that is antiseptic, flexible, and waterproof, while letting the skin breathe. The one-ounce size is small and convenient. Clean the skin, spray or coat, and let dry. A second coating may be added for additional protection. Keep toes bent when applying and drying. There is no residue or stickiness. Do not apply to infected or draining sites. It is strong smelling stuff, so use with good ventilation and avoid breathing too deeply. Its main ingredients are pyroxylin solution, acetone ACS, oil of cloves, and 8-hydroxyquinoline. Look for New-Skin at drug stores. For more information contact Medtech Laboratories Inc.

Rubbing Alcohol   Renown walker Colin Fletcher suggests using rubbing alcohol on feet as a skin toughener.[12] Use it on your toes, soles, and heels several times daily. While walking and hiking with sore feet, he uses almost hourly applications of rubbing alcohol followed by foot powder. Rubbing alcohol is available in most drug stores.

Tincture of Benzoin   Tincture of benzoin is available in either liquid, swabs, or squeeze vials. Commonly used as a tape or bandage adherent, it is sometimes used as a skin toughener. After applying the tincture, let it dry for about three minutes before applying tape. Tincture of benzoin leaves an orange-brownish color on the skin. Avoid getting the tincture into any cuts, abrasions, or open blisters — it can burn! Usually available in a liquid at drug stores, pharmacies, or medical supply stores. The swabs or squeeze vials may require a special order.

Tom Crawford's Tea and Betadine® Skin Toughener

Tom Crawford is an ultrarunner who has completed numerous ultras including the challenging Death Valley to Mt. Whitney ultra both one way and as an out-and-back run. Tom's method begins with mixing ten Lipton tea bags and one cup of Betadine into 1/2 gallon of water. For one week, dip your feet 20 times over the course of a day, letting them air dry between dips. The second week, add one cup of salt to the water, tea, and Betadine mixture. Then for one week, soak your feet for 20 minutes at a time, several times daily. Betadine can be found in drug stores and medical supply stores.

Richard Benyo recalled how he used Tom's method to prepare his feet for the Death Valley 300. "Each night I'd pour the solution into a plastic foot bath and keep my soles and toes in the solution for fifteen minutes; then I'd alternately raise one foot out of the brew for three minutes, allowing it to dry, then lower it and bring the other foot out. I'd do that for a half-hour. Then I'd let them dry and I'd go to bed with orange soles. When I showered the next morning, it would wash off. But little by little, it made my feet more resistant to blisters."[13] Even with this preparation, Richard sometimes found his feet often susceptible to blisters.

12

Taping for Blisters

If your feet are prone to blistering, taping may be a lifesaver. After 12 hours of a 72-hour run, my Vaseline-coated feet were almost too sore to run on, and I had a blister between two toes. Nancy Crawford, an experienced running friend, taught me how to prepare my feet for taping and use duct tape to both fix the blister and tape the tender balls of my feet which would likely blister in the hours ahead. I completed the next 60 hours without a foot problem! While you may consider duct taping an extreme, consider the benefits of taping if you are highly susceptible to blisters. You can tape before your event as a proactive preventative measure or in a reactive mode after hot spots or blisters develop.

Taping Basics

There are several types of tape available to try.

- ☞ Duct tape is a 2″ wide, very sticky silver tape with a fabric core that has excellent adhesive qualities. Duct tape is available at any hardware store.
- ☞ Elastikon™ from Johnson & Johnson Medical Inc. is a medium-thickness elastic porous tape which comes in 1″, 2″, 3″, and 4″ widths.
- ☞ 3M's Medipore™ is a thin, soft knit-style tape which comes in

1″, 2″, 3″, and 4″ widths and is perforated in easy-to-tear strips. This tape conforms nicely to the contours of the feet.

☞ 3M's Microfoam™ is a 1/32″ thick, soft foam tape which comes in a 1″, 2″, and 4″ widths.

The Johnson & Johnson's Elastikon and 3M's Medipore and Microfoam tapes can be found at or ordered through most medical supply stores.

Runners who decide to try taping should purchase a tape adherent which provides a taping base to hold the tape to the skin. The best adherents are Cramer Products' Tuf-Skin or Mueller's Tuffner Clear Spray, both a colorless spray or the brownish tincture of benzoin in a liquid or swabs. (See the chapter *Skin Toughener and Tape Adherents* on page 63). These products help the tape adhere to the skin. Remember to let the tape adherent dry before applying the tape. After spraying and taping your feet, be sure to apply a sprinkling of powder to the sprayed areas that are not taped to counteract any adhesive left uncovered.

Preparation includes several steps. Before taping, clean the feet of their natural oils, dust, and dirt. Rubbing alcohol works well to clean the feet and dries quickly. For fanny pack use, buy alcohol wipes in small disposable packets. Next apply the tape adherent to the areas needing taping and let dry. Then apply the tape based on your specific needs or problems.

Keep the tape as smooth as possible. Ridges in the tape may cut into the skin and lead to irritation which may cause blisters. If the tape must be overlapped, be sure the overlapping edge of the tape is in the same direction as the force of motion. For example, if taping the ball of the foot, the force is towards the rear of the foot, so the most forward piece of tape should overlap over the piece towards the back. If taping the heel, the force is towards the rear and up the back of the heel, so the tape on the bottom of the heel should overlap the piece higher up on the back of the heel. This will keep the tape from catching on the sock and peeling up. The less overlap the better. Applying the tape too tight may cause circulation problems. If, after application, the skin becomes discolored, cool, or numb, loosen the tape.

Place a single layer of toilet paper or tissue over any existing blisters where the outer skin has pulled loose from the inner skin. This keeps the adhesive from attacking the sensitive area and protects the blistered skin when the tape is removed. You can also substitute a piece of duct tape for the tissue, sticky side to sticky side. This allows the slick side of the duct tape to face the hot spot or blister.

After the foot is taped, several finishing touches should be made. Run a thin layer of Bag Balm, Vaseline or similar lubricant over the tape and around the edges. This reinforces the tape's status as part of your foot by providing a barrier that neutralizes any adhesive leaks and allows the taped surface to slip easily across friction points without snagging. Finally use a lubricant or powder on your feet to cut the sticky pre-tape base, if one was used.

You may be able to tape all areas of your feet yourself. If you have problems reaching the outer edges of your feet, your heels, or any other awkward area, find someone to help with the taping.

When removing the duct tape, work slowly and carefully. You would not want to pull off a layer of skin or a toenail with the tape. Work from the sides to the center, using the fingers of one hand to hold the skin while pulling the tape with the other hand. Ultrarunner Suzi Thibeault suggests using baby oil and gentle massage to roll off the tape and excessive adhesive.

Taping is useful for pre-run preparation as well as to fix newly developed problem spots. If you typically blister on the balls of your feet, consider taping before the run when you have the time to do it right rather then at an aid station when you need every minute of time. Practice taping to learn how best to apply the tape to meet your particular needs. Determine how much time is needed to do a complete application. If you are going to have crew support for an event, teach them how to do the taping.

Below are two methods of taping the feet. The first uses duct tape. The second uses Johnson & Johnson Elastikon tape. Each method can be used with the other types of tape mentioned earlier. If you are bothered by blisters, and powders and/or lubricants do not work, try the different tapes to find a tape and taping method which works for you. In the chapter *Foot Care Kits* on page 153, you will find a list of taping materials to carry during your runs and hikes.

Duct Tape Techniques

Duct tape is tough. A mail order catalog offers a T-shirt with a picture of the familiar silver roll and the words "When the Going Gets Tough, The Tough Use Duct Tape." Ultrarunner Ivy Franklin blistered so badly at the Arkansas Traveller 100 in 1994 that she dropped at 68 miles. Then she learned about the miracle of duct taping and ran the Umstead Trail 100 in 1995 and returned to the Arkansas Traveller 100 in 1996 without either blisters or hot spots.

Many runners have successfully used Gary Cantrell's article "From the South: The Amazing Miracle of Duct Tape"[14] to learn how to prevent and treat blisters. Gary's basic principle is to cover the spot that's injured with a patch and in some cases then anchor the edges and corners of that patch. The powerful adhesive of duct tape holds it true to the outline of your skin and the tough, plastic outer tape skin reinforced with fabric can withstand almost unlimited friction. The friction points on your skin will then have an additional layer of skin — the duct tape. Gary's method follows, with a few of my time-tested additions.

Remember a few general duct tape rules. Choose a good quality duct tape with a visible fabric core, not a plastic cheap imitation. Many hardware stores carry several types of duct tape. The standard grade is typically nine-millimeters thick while the contractor and professional grades are generally ten-millimeters thick. Duct tape is only available in a 2″ width. You may find it called "Duct Tape" or "Duck$_{Brand}$ Tape." Although the tape is sometimes available in a variety of colors the common silver tape works the best.

The tape is applied over the danger spots where blisters frequently occur. Don't apply tape where it is not needed. Use only a single thickness since additional layers become too hard and unyielding. When the tape is applied, that part of the foot should be flexed to its maximum extension. Cut the ends of the tape so they are rounded. If your feet are hairy, shave the parts where the tape will be applied.

Taping the ball of the foot   Take a long strip of full-width tape and place it, adhesive side up, on the floor. Place your foot on it at a right angle, with the trouble spot dead center on the tape. Then flatten your foot to make it as wide as possible and pull the ends of the tape up, either overlapping them on the top of your foot or cutting them an inch up on either side of the foot. Cut the tape at the forward edge of the ball of the foot so it does not contact or cut into the crease at the base of the toes or the toes themselves.

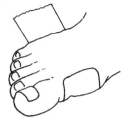

Cut tape to conform to the
shape of the forefoot

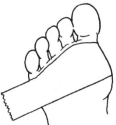

Wrap tape up the sides
of the foot

Taping the toes   First tear off a small strip and use it to wrap from the base of the toenail around the tip of the toe and to the bottom of the toe even with the end on top, leaving two free ends. (Omit this step for toes that don't blister at the tip.) Wrap another strip around the circumference of the toe, covering the free ends of the first strip, if it was used. Overlap them slightly on top of the toe. Always use a large enough strip to cover the toe's "knuckle joint" so that both outside edges are too small to slide over the joint and cause the tape to bunch off or slip off the end of the toe. Never extend the edge far enough down that it will dig into the tender skin between the toes. For taping against toenail friction, tape the receiving toe, rather than the offending nail.

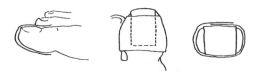

Use two pieces of tape for toes, one from top to
bottom over the tip and another around the toe

Taping between toe and foot   Cut a small pad of sterile gauze or tissue and place it firmly over the blister. Fasten it in place with a slightly larger square of tape. Take a long thin strip of tape and run it diagonally, corner to corner, between your toes from the top of your foot to the ball of your foot. Take another long, thin strip and do the same with the two remaining corners. Now you have a pad on the blister, the pad protected by duct tape, and the whole thing held firmly in place by the four strips attaching the corners to the tops and bottoms of your feet. Now anchor these strips with the single piece described for the ball of the foot, and the most difficult blister of all is fixed.

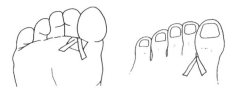

Two diagonal strips of tape anchors the patch over a blister

Taping the bottom of the heel   Start with a large patch of tape covering the entire heel. Attach it with both the foot and ankle flexed forward and up (pull your toes toward your shin). Take a long strip of tape cut to a 1″ width and cover the forward edge of the patch under your foot and bring the ends up to overlap on top of the foot. Take another medium strip and cover the edge on the back of your heel and bring the ends around the ankle to overlap on top of the first strip.

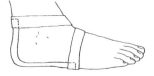

Tape under the foot, up the heel, and secure it with two strips around the foot

Suzi T's Taping Technique

Suzi Thibeault, an ultrarunner, developed this taping technique while completing the Grand Slam of trail ultrarunning, five 100-mile runs in one summer with only a couple of small "tape" blisters. Suzi stresses this technique will not work for everybody. Your individual footprint and running style may affect the taping. Suzi's technique involves taping the bottom of each foot up to the heel, around the sides of the foot, and each toe. She tapes the night before an event after taking a shower. She has often had the tape on up to 36 hours without a problem.

Suzi uses Johnson & Johnson's Elastikon tape in 2″ and 4″ widths. River and stream crossings are not a problem since the tape is porous and dries as fast as socks and shoes. Do not stretch the tape, simply form it to the foot and press firmly. All points where the tape folds or is pinched together should be folded like a gift wrap fold and cut flush with the skin. This is truly preventative maintenance, creating a sock type effect. Determine your specific hot spot or blister problems and try taping as needed. When cutting the tape flush with the skin, be careful not to cut the skin. She recommends baby oil and gentle massage to remove the tape.

Suzi uses the following three steps to tape the whole foot. If you only have problems on the ball of the foot, the heel, or the toes, use the appropriate taping strategy.

Taping the bottom of the foot   Apply a 4″ piece of tape from just behind the bend of the toe base, centering the tape on the bottom of the foot from front to back. Have equal edges on the inside and outside of the foot. Trim the front edge to follow the contour of the toe base avoiding the crease. Bring the back edge up the heel and fold over on each side, like a gift wrap, making a dart. Cut the fold flush with the foot, leaving two edges just meeting in a "V" pattern.

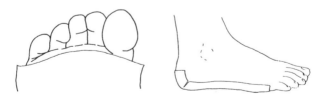

Center the tape on the foot to allow equal amounts up the sides of the foot, cut to the shape of the forefoot, and mold up the heel

Taping the sides of the foot Once the 4″ piece is in place on the bottom of the foot, apply a 2″ piece around the foot from one side to the other. Slightly overlap over the edge of the 4″ tape. Trim the edges to avoid rubbing at the toe crease and ankle bone. If you find the bottom edge of the tape catching on your socks, put this layer on before taping the bottom of the foot. Then tape the bottom of the foot so that tape overlaps the side of the foot tape. This method keeps the overlapping tape in the direction of the force of motion as described earlier.

Apply a single strip of tape around the back of the heel, overlapping the bottom of the foot piece

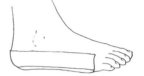

Taping the toes Toes are taped with pieces of the 2″ tape. Tape only the last two joints, avoiding the crease at the base of the toes. Roll the tape around the toe, over-lapping over the toenails for a double-layer but keeping a single-layer on the sides of the toes. Fold the excess over at the tips of the toes, pinching the top and bottom together. Cut the tape flush with the skin, leaving no overlap.

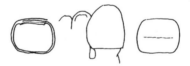

Tape toes with one piece around the toe, pinch it closed and cut it flush with the skin

13

Orthotics

Many runners wear an orthotic device in one or both shoes which helps maintain the foot in a functionally correct position. Support can be provided for flatfeet and pronation problems. Malalignment problems such as leg length inequality can be corrected. They can also relieve pressure by providing support behind a problem area as in a callous, neuroma, or metatarsal injury. Typically prescribed by a podiatrist or orthopedist, orthotics are medical devices made from cast impressions of your feet. A properly fit orthotic will control arch and pressure point problems.

Orthotics may be soft, semi-rigid, or rigid, and are made specifically for your feet. They may be made in the office from common materials or custom made of special materials. Materials may include felt pads, cork, viscoelastic, silicon, closed-cell rubber or closed-cell polyethylene. Orthotics can be made in various lengths and include metatarsal pads or heel wedges. They are made to work in partnership with your boots and shoes. Poor-quality boots and shoes may alter the corrective action of an orthotic.

In the article "The Ideal Running Orthosis: A Philosophy of Design,"[15] the authors build a case for the ideal orthotic. They recommend a custom fit in either semi-rigid or flexible design, light-weight, yet inexpensive, with a covering to decrease shear while giving control to both the forefoot and hindfoot, all while retaining memory in its shape and being adjustable at a later time. It also needs to be transferable to most of the client's shoes. They place orthotics in two categories of design: corrective and accommodative. A corrective orthotic should attempt, with a rigid design, to correct the foot's position so that its abnormal anatomy will mold to the corrected position. An accommodative orthotic should attempt to relieve areas of high stress or reposition the foot to better deal with its stress, usually with a soft or semi-rigid design.

Your podiatrist or orthopedist can ask the right questions and order the right tests to make the correct diagnosis of which type of corrective orthotic is necessary. The typical process includes a detailed injury history, complete lower-extremity biomechanical examination including a gait analysis, and a check of your shoes or boots. The aim is to identify the cause of your injury and try to prevent its continuation or recurrence. Orthotics may be prescribed for the treatment of plantar fasciitis, tendinitis, runner's knee, shin splints, lower back pain, and other conditions. Patient compliance in wearing the orthotic is the dominate issue in resolving foot problems. Modifications to the orthotics may be necessary to ensure a proper fit. If the orthotic is uncomfortable it will not be worn. Your podiatrist or orthopedist will provide instructions on use and care of your orthotics.

Talk to your podiatrist or orthopedist about what you need to do to help the orthotics work. He or she may give you a detailed treatment schedule of stretching and strengthening exercises and advice on shoe or boot selection. You may also be advised to wear the orthotics for several hours a day and gradually work your way up to longer periods.

If your foot seems to slip on your orthotic, ask about changing the surface material. A thin layer of Spenco insole material or your favorite insole material can usually be glued to the orthotic using rubber cement.

Mail order orthotics need to be checked out thoroughly and purchased only through reputable companies. Adjustments to mail order orthotics can be difficult. Avoid drug store orthotics. Arch supports sold in sporting goods and drug stores should not be mistaken for orthotics. The Hapad, Lynco, and Spenco orthotics identified below are just three of many low cost orthotics which can be helpful as an alternative to custom orthotics and "quick-fix" drug store remedies.

Nick Williams had "... tried hard orthotics, soft orthotics, Spenco orthotics, and just about anything else to keep my feet from hurting." Then an orthopedic surgeon told him about Hapads and gave him a pair. They have kept him pain free for the last five years and are flexible on trails. Nick now swears by Hapads and via e-mail told Ed Furtaw about them. Ed wore custom made orthotics for 10 years but now uses the Comf-Orthotic 3/4-length insoles, without heel pain, saying "They are definitely more comfortable than wearing orthotics." Ed added the Hapad Scaphoid Pads for extra arch support. Now Ed's wife has switched from custom orthotics to the Comf-Orthotic. After an area on one arch got a little sore, they peeled away some of the wool material to make it fit better. Ed believes that "With something like Hapads, a person can take more responsibility for their own orthotic adjustments, which would be very difficult or impossible with custom-molded rigid orthotics." An orthopedist told me that if he had only one product to offer his patients, he would choose Hapads!

Hapad Comf-Orthotic   Hapad makes several orthotics which are popular because of their low cost and effectiveness. The 3/4-length and full-length insoles are helpful for heel spur pain and flat feet. The 3-Way Heel/Arch/Metatarsal Insole is a combination longitudinal metatarsal arch pad with a heel extension and is effective for plantar fasciitis. These three are made from coiled, spring-like wool fibers which provide firm and resilient support as they mold and shape to the foot. The full-length contoured Comf-Orthotic Sports Replacement Insole is made in three layers with a moisture-wicking suede top, a ventilated Poron® middle layer for shock absorption, and a bottom of Microcel® "Puff," a self-molding footbed. The insole includes a metatarsal bar to relieve pressure at the ball of the foot, a medial arch support to limit pronation, and a heel cup for stability and control of the foot and ankle. For more information contact Hapad, Inc.

Lynco® Biomechanical Orthotic Systems   Apex offers the Lynco Biomechanical Orthotic System, a "ready-made" triple-density orthotic system that comes in enough variations to accommodate 90% of foot disorders. By identifying your foot type as either normal, high arched, or flat/over pronated, a model is determined. Three basic models are offered: 1) heel pain related to heel spurs, heel pain syndrome, Achilles tendinitis, and plantar fasciitis; 2) arch pain related to arch strain, post-tib tendinitis, and plantar fasciitis; and 3) metatarsal pain related to metatarsalgia, Morton's toe, and Morton's neuroma. Each model, based on foot type, comes with either a neutral-cupped heel or a medial posted heel, and with or without a metatarsal pad. Additional Reflex™ self-adhesive pads can be added to the orthotics to relieve pain from Morton's toe, sesamoiditis, and leg-length discrepancy. These orthotics are a superb alternative to custom-made orthotics. For more information contact Apex Foot Health Industries, Inc.

Spenco Orthotic Arch Support   Spenco makes an Orthotic Arch Support which is heated in water and then shaped to your foot. They are available in either 3/4- or full-length. For more information contact Spenco.

14

Nutrition for the Feet

In order to keep our feet healthy it is necessary to take care of them and to give them the nutrition they need. But then how many of us know what our feet really need?

Jillian Standish, a certified massage therapist, feels many runners simply don't think about using lotions or creams on their feet. Most of her clients are average runners who need the benefits of massage to enhance their running. Jillian focuses part of her massages on the feet since the lower leg muscles attach into the feet. As a pre-race conditioner, the massage helps loosen the muscles, often lengthening the runner's stride. As a post-race conditioner, she massages knots out of tired and stressed muscles.

In the summer when we are most active, our feet are often abused. Our feet become hard and callused or blistered by our multi-day hikes, long training runs on back-to-back days, cross-sport training, going barefoot, or wearing sandals without socks. We repeatedly stress our feet without giving them time to recover and to heal. In dry and cold weather our skin easily becomes too dry, resulting in cracks in the skin. When these cracks are deep they are called fissures and are often accompanied by calluses.

Use creams or lotions which help improve the skin's texture and tone by exfoliating dry and dead skin and allow newly rejuvenated skin to emerge. Some creams contain Alpha Hydroxy Acids which are all-natural substances found in fruits and sugar cane which generally speed up the exfoliation process. Ultrarunner Roy Pirrung uses flax oil products to keep his skin well conditioned.

Long distance hiker Brick Robbins finds that after several months on the trail he has a hard time with "stuff" growing on his feet. He has solved this common problem by soaking his feet for 20 minutes in a solution of about a gallon of water and two to four ounces of providone-iodine every week or so. It keeps his "... feet from smelling too bad and seemed to kill the stuff that had started to grow under one of my big toes." Betadine will also work as an alternative to providone-iodine.

Home Health   Home Health Products For Life makes a complete line of skin care products. Products for the feet include two Podiatrist's Secret™ products: Total Foot Recovery™ a cream/lotion with Alpha Hydroxy Acid and deep-penetrating Urethin™ to soften dry and callused feet, and Callus Treatment Cream with Urethin to break down painful, hardened skin. Both products leave your feet softer and smoother. For ordering information, contact Home Health.

A wide assortment of products are readily available at your local health food store or drug store. Below is a sampling of some products. Check your health food store or drug store for additional skin care products.

☞ FootTherapy® Natural Mineral Foot Bath can be used to soak and soften corns and calluses.

☞ Flaxseed oil products containing sources of essential fatty acids for proper skin conditioning.

☞ Peppermint Foot Lotion is a cooling lotion containing Chinese peppermint oil with arnica.

☞ Bioforce of America makes A. Vogel's Homeopathic 7 Herb Cream, a combination of herbs and oils in a natural base formulated to soften and smooth rough, dry, or cracked skin.

15

Hydration, Dehydration, and Sodium

A subject often overlooked is the effect of dehydration and the loss of important electrolytes to the skin. Long periods of physical exercise cause stress to the extremities as fluid accumulates in the hands and feet. Fingers and toes often swell as they retain fluid because of low sodium. This causes foot problems as the soft, water-logged tissues become vulnerable to the rubbing and pounding as we continue to run and hike. Make sure that you replace electrolytes, especially on long events. Drinking water or even sports drinks may not provide the proper replacement of sodium and other important electrolytes.

It is important to understand, as ultrarunner Jay Hodde notes, "... 'proper hydration' and 'well hydrated' should not be used interchangeably. Being well hydrated with fluids says nothing about the sodium content of the fluid; both are important." As extra fluid accumulates in the tissues of the feet, from being well hydrated yet having low sodium, the likelihood of blister formation increases. When you become fluid-deficient, the skin loses its normal levels of water in the skin and loses its turgor. Then it easily rubs or folds over on itself which leads to blisters. The use of a sodium replacement product in prolonged physical activity can help in the prevention of blisters. SUCCEED! Electrolyte Caps and Thermotabs are two products helpful in maintaining hydration and proper sodium levels.

SUCCEED! Electrolyte Caps   Ultrarunner and race director Karl King developed the SUCCEED! Electrolyte Caps to provide electrolytes that are commonly found in blood plasma, in the proper proportions for hours of exercise. The caps contain a chemical buffering system of sodium chloride, sodium bicarbonate, sodium citrate, sodium phosphate, and potassium chloride, that neutralizes the acids formed during heavy exercise. This both reduces nausea associated with exercise, particularly in the heat, and reduces swelling of hands and feet typically common after many hours of exercise. Karl reports positive results with the caps — a reduction in hot spots and blisters and reduced swelling in the hands and feet. SUCCEED! Electrolyte Caps are designed for those engaging in physical activities which make them sweat heavily. They should not be used when water is in short supply. For information contact UltraFit.

Thermotabs®   Thermotabs are buffered salt tablets which can be taken to prevent muscle cramps or heat prostration due excessive perspiration. Its active ingredients are sodium chloride and potassium chloride. Look for Thermotabs at your local drug store or pharmacy. Thermotabs are made by Menley & James Laboratories, Inc.

16

Anti-Perspirants
for the Feet

Some individuals have problems with excessive perspiration on their feet. The medical term "hyperhidrosis" refers to excessive moisture. This moisture often increases the chance of blisters. In these individuals, the use of an anti-perspirant on the feet may reduce the formation of blisters. Two main products offer a solution to this problem.

Foot Solution   ONOX Inc. makes Foot Solution, a spray solution made to control excessive moisture and foot odor. A combination of mineral salts decreases excessive sweat and foot odor symptoms. The spray also helps reduce blistering and itching while repelling athlete's foot fungus. Ingredients include zinc chloride, deionized water, sodium chloride, sodium nitrate, boric acid, and sodium silco-fluoride. Be aware that the salt solution will sting if you have cuts or breaks in your skin. Foot Solution is available in a four-ounce spray pump. ONOX also offers two products for relief from poison oak: Clean-Off to remove oils and Itch Relief to relieve itching caused by plants and insects. Foot Solution, with its sodium concentrations, also works on poison oak. For more information contact ONOX Inc.

Gordon's #5™   Gordon Laboratories makes Gordon's #5, an aerosol foot powder which is helpful in reducing foot perspiration and foot odor. Gordon's #5 is available in a four-ounce size. Available only by special order through your local drug store, pharmacy, or podiatrist from Gordon Laboratories.

17

Gaiters

In 1989, before my third Western States 100 Mile Endurance Run, I knew I had to do something extra to help my feet. Since I was prone to blisters and the trail was known for its dust and rocks, I decided to make a pair of gaiters. My home-made gaiters are described below. While I realize the gaiters alone did not make the whole difference, I did lower my personal best time by 1 1/2 hours. The bottom line was that my feet were protected from the dust, grit, and rocks of the trail, and I had minimal problems.

Gaiters have proven themselves as functional trail running gear that all dedicated trail runners should have in their equipment bag. Hikers wearing low-top boots should consider the benefits of gaiters. Forming a barrier around the leg and the top of the shoe, gaiters keep

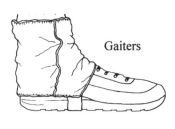

Gaiters

rocks, dust, and water-borne grit from getting into socks or between the socks and shoe. Gaiters can mean the difference between finishing a trail run or long hike with feet in good shape or feet plagued with hot spots and blisters. Most gaiters close on the side or in the front with Velcro™. There are four main sources for gaiters.

Homemade Gaiters　　Homemade gaiters for running shoes or boots can be made out of a pair of regular white crew socks.

Pull the socks on your feet and with a scissors, cut the socks around the foot at the top of the shoe line. Toss out the foot portions. Fold the top of the sock down on itself so the folded down top covers the top of the shoe. Make a small hole in this folded down top at the back of the shoe and just to the rear of each upper shoe lace eyelet. Make similar holes in the shoe. Through the shoe hole place a plastic twist tie from a loaf of bread or similar package. By twisting the ties through these matching holes you have effectively covered the top of the shoes. Undo the twist ties to change shoes or socks while leaving the sock gaiter on your leg.

Outdoor Research   Outdoor Research makes three gaiter styles appropriate for running and hiking. The Flex-Tex™ Low Gaiter is a one-size-fits-all. Made from stretchy Spandura fabric, these have an eyelet on either side for a lace which goes under the shoe's arch. These gaiters are suited for hiking boots or running shoes. The Rocky Mountain High™ Gaiters are available in either Gore-Tex fabric or packcloth in small, medium, large, and extra-large. The Rocky Mountain Low™ Gaiters are made from vapor permeable uncoated packcloth in one-size-fits-all. For more information contact Outdoor Research.

Trail Gators™   Trail Gators are a running shoe gaiter designed by Jim O'Brien, a veteran ultrarunner. Jim's gaiters come in several sizes and a combination of colors. Made from quick drying and breathable Supplex nylon, these gaiters have a nylon strap which goes under the shoe's arch. Sizes are medium, men's shoe size, 6-9.5, and large, 10-13. Small and extra large are available by special order. These could be used on mid- and low-top hiking boots by lengthening the strap as show below. When the nylon strap wears out, change the strap by following the instructions below or purchase a new pair of gaiters. For more information contact Trail Gaitors.

Western States 100 Trail Gaiters   Norm Klein, Race Director of the Western States 100 Mile Endurance Run, offers running shoe trail gaiters. These gaiters are made of nylon Condura fabric with a light urethane coating. A snap on each side of the gaiter attaches to the nylon strap that goes under the shoe and is also held in place with a Velcro strip. An extra pair of straps is included with each pair of gaiters. These gaiters are available in medium, large, and extra-large sizes. These gaiters can be worn with many of the low-top hiking boots either as is or by lengthening the strap. For more information contact Norm Klein.

Repairing Gaiter Straps   The nylon straps which go under the shoes and boots will wear out over time as the trails and rocks take their toll. Wrapping the straps with duct tape can help extend their life span, but they will wear out. There are two ways to replace the worn out straps.

The first method simply uses 1/4″ nylon cord. Cut the old strap 3/4″ from its attachment to the gaiter. Use a lighted match to slightly melt the ends of the straps to prevent fraying. Be careful to not touch the melted nylon until it cools. Punch a small hole in the middle of the 3/4″ section and use another lighted match to slightly melt the edges of the hole. Thread the nylon cord through the holes and knot securely so the length is the same as the old strap. Slightly melt the ends of the cord to avoid fraying.

The second method, recommended by ultrarunner Kirk Boisseree, actually replaces the strap itself with the following materials which are usually found in fabric stores: 1″ wide nylon webbing, size 24 (5/8″) large snaps (four sets of male and female pieces), and a snap installation tool. The snap tool can usually be found in craft or sewing stores. Make the new straps as follows:

1. Using the old strap as a guide, cut two pieces of webbing the length of the old strap.
2. At each end of the replacement straps, install a female snap. Use a center punch or a nail to make a hole in the center of the strap 3/4″ from each end. Push the snap through the hole and set the snap using the tool and following the instructions on the package. Repeat for all four snaps, making sure the snaps face the same way on each strap end.
3. Install the male snaps on the old straps about 1/2″ to 3/4″ from the gaiter. Using the center punch and installation tool, center the male snap in the hole, facing the outside of the shoe and set the snap.
4. Cut the center out of the worn strap by cutting about 1/2″ from the new snaps.

5. Use a lighted match to slightly melt the ends of the straps to prevent fraying. Be careful to not touch the melted nylon until it cools.
6. Snap on the new straps and check for a proper fit.

18

Lacing Options

Some runners have problems with laces causing friction and pressure. After a long run or hike, some runners and hikers experience bruising over the instep where the laces tie. Laces can be adjusted to fine tune the fit of the shoe or boot and to relieve pressure over the instep. The lacing variations described below can make a shoe fit better and allow for needed spacing in the tongue area or provide for better heel control. The conventional method of lacing, criss-cross to the top of the shoe, works best for the majority of people. In the illustrations, dotted lines show where laces are hidden from view.

Flat feet, high arches or not enough support in the arches, narrow or wide feet, and heel control problems can be helped, to varying degrees, by lacing techniques. Several of the lacing techniques described below work best with shoes having alternating eyelets spaced apart, not up and down in a straight line.

For narrow feet, use the eyelets farthest from the tongue of the shoe. This will bring up the sides of the shoe for a tighter fit across the top of the foot. This method works on shoes with variable width eyelets.

For wide feet, use the eyelets closest to the tongue of the shoe. This gives the foot more space by giving more width across the lace area. This method works best on shoes with variable width eyelets.

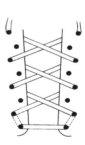

Narrow feet

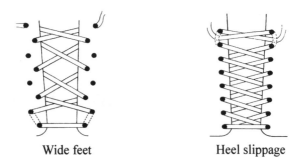

Wide feet   Heel slippage

For heel slippage or problems, use every eyelet, making sure that the area closest to the heel is tied tightly while less tension is used near the toes. When you have reached the next to the last eyelet on each side, thread the lace through the top eyelet of the same side, making a small loop. Then thread the opposite lace through each opposite loop before tying the laces together at the top.

High arches can be helped by lacing the shoes so the laces go straight across. After lacing the bottom two eyelets on the outer side to the inner two eyelets, lace up two eyelets on the same inner side and cross over to the outer side. Lace through these two eyelets and move up two eyelets on the same outer side. Continue this alternating method until one set of eyelets is left. Now lace up to the top eyelets on each side.

An alternative method for high arches is to lace one lace through the first two bottom eyelets and then every other eyelet to the top. A second lace is threaded through the remaining eyelets. This allows tighter lacing at the ball of the foot and the ankle while the mid-foot is laced looser. With this method, quick adjustments are easily made for uphills and downhills.

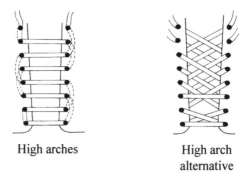

High arches   High arch
                                                  alternative

For a narrow heel and wide forefoot use one pair of laces per shoe. Lace one through the bottom half of the eyelets tied loosely. Lace the other through the top half of the eyelets tied more tightly than the bottom lace.

For foot pain, lace as normal for your foot type and skip the eyelets over the pain area.

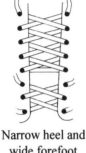

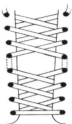

Narrow heel and
wide forefoot

Foot pain

For toenail problems or corns, lace down from the top eyelet opposite the problem toe to the bottom eyelet on the side of the problem toe, leaving enough end to tie the laces together. Then from the bottom up, side-to-side until the top eyelet is reached. This method creates an upward tension on the bottom eyelet over the problem toe, relieving pressure.

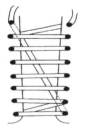

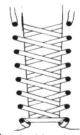

Toenail problems or corns

Constant toe pressure

To maintain a consistent lace pressure at the toes, lace the bottom eyelets as usual. Then lock the lace in place by looping the lace around and back through the same eyelet. Continue lacing as normal. The technique can be modified by locking the lace at the second or third eyelet. This allows you to tie the laces as tight as you want above the lock while keeping the laces as loose as desired below the lock.

Several lacing products are worth considering for running shoes and some boots. These products replace the normal shoelaces and end the problem of laces coming untied or broken. Experiment with stretch laces to find the most comfortable degree of lace tightness which does not cause undo pressure on the instep and yet controls the heel. A product which can help with instep irritations is a tongue cushion.

Coilers™   These easy to use shoelaces are fabric-covered permanently-coiled elastic. The laces are twisted through the eyelets and pulled to the desired pressure. The laces can be tightened or loosened as necessary. Originally designed for tri-athletes, they can be used on shoe or mid- and low-top boots with up to eight pair of eyelets. Coilers are available in a variety of colors. For more information contact Allor Medical Inc.

Hapad Tongue Cushion   Hapad makes a Tongue Cushion which prevents rubbing and comforts shoe irritations at the instep. If you have narrow heels, it also holds the foot back into the heel of the shoe for a better fit. The coiled, spring-like wool fibers provide firm and resilient support. The pad attaches to the underside of the tongue of the shoe. For more information contact Hapad, Inc.

InterLace® Shoe Laces   InterLace shoelaces are made for all types of footwear. The laces are made of a thin, stretchy vinyl tube. The laces are fed through the shoe eyelets from the top to the bottom and joined at the bottom with a connector. This allows you to slide on your shoes or mid- and low-top boots. There are no knots or bows. These laces eliminate the problem of pressure on the foot where the shoelace knots. InterLaces are available in a variety of colors and sizes. They may not work for high-top shoes or boots. For more information contact the InterLace Corporation.

Willy's Easy Laces   Easy Laces are an alternative to shoelaces for running shoes and most hiking boots. The lace is a stretchy elastic cord with an interlocking lock where the usual bow is tied. The foot is slipped into the shoe or boot without releasing the lock, or the lock can be released to open the shoe further. The laces are available in 20″, 30″, 60″ lengths and in a myriad of colors. Easy Laces are made by the Stretch-Lace Company. For more information contact Kayne & Co.

19

Changing Your
Shoes and Socks

On long runs, determine how often you will change your shoes and socks. Ultrarunner Dave Scott changes his shoes four to five times in a 100-mile trail race. At each change he reapplies more Vaseline to his toes. Aid stations that are accessible to crew support or aid stations that have your drop bags are the best choices. When possible, change your socks and/or shoes before problems develop. Dry skin is more resistant to blister formation than skin that has been softened by moisture. Trail runs and hiking often make for wet shoes and boots which become dirt-caked. Shoes and socks should be changed as soon as possible after getting wet. Depending on the event, you may choose to change at pre-determined points or pre-determined times. This may be as many as four to five times in a long, 100-mile run. At these times, the feet should be inspected for problems and treatments made.

While shoes and socks do dry out after a stream crossing or in rain, continuing to run or hike may cause the skin on your feet to become overly soft and tender and more prone to blisters. Softening of the skin, called maceration, can cause skin over and around blisters to separate. Where the blister is already ruptured, the skin then opens up. When the skin has been wet for long periods of time, it is not uncommon, when removing socks, to find the skin as shriveled as a prune and the skin separating. The use of high-technology oversocks to keep the feet dry can help reduce maceration and blisters. Refer to the *High-Technology Oversocks* section on page 52 for information on these socks.

As difficult as it becomes, you must take the time to properly manage your feet, or your feet will manage you as problems develop and you are reduced to a slow, limping walk. When you are close to an age-group win, a personal best, simply finishing within the time limit, or reaching a specific trail destination, the three to ten minutes necessary for foot care may seem like a lifetime. Only you can make the decision on taking the time to care for your feet. I have seen many runners take off their shoes and socks to reveal skin which fall off the bottom of their feet. Not small pieces but enough to cover half their foot! It cannot be emphasized enough — take the time necessary to manage your feet or they will manage you.

Runners may choose to carry an extra pair of socks and a small foot care kit in a fanny pack, allowing for road or trailside foot care as necessary. Hikers need to carry a footcare kit as part of a first-aid kit. They should wash their dirty socks daily and dry them on the back of their packs.

In extremely cold weather, it is important to keep the feet dry and warm. Socks and footwear which are too tight can cause constriction and impede circulation. Changing from wet into dry socks helps keep the feet warm. The use of moisture-wicking socks also is helpful. See the section *High-Technology Oversocks* on page 52 for information on these socks which can help ward off cold.

Frostbite can happen to toes. An understanding of frostbite can help runners and hikers avoid it. Frostbite requires freezing temperature. Tight shoes, socks, and shoe laces can cause constriction. Dehydration makes athletes more susceptible to frostbite. The use of anti-perspirants to control moisture can help. Symptoms of frostbite include cold, pain, dulling of the pain (frostnip), numbness, a doughy or wooden look, and pain on rewarming. If you suspect frostbite, do not wash away the skin's natural oils. If your feet are frostbitten, do not rewarm them if you must walk to help, but wait until medical help is available.

20

Crew Support for Ultradistance Events

If you will be participating in an event where you have crew support to help you at aid stations, make sure to discuss foot care issues with them before the event. Let them know if there will be shoe or sock changes at particular aid stations, and if so, what specific shoes or socks you will want. Let them know all of the following.

☞ How to take your shoes and socks off to avoid making any foot problems worse.

☞ How to put new shoes and socks back on.

☞ What powders and/or lubricants you use and where on your feet you use them.

☞ How tight you like your shoes tied, and whether you use single or double knots.

☞ How you want to deal with hot spots, blisters, toenails, or other unique problems.

Practice this with your crew at home, well in advance of the run. Find what works and what doesn't work. It is important to know how much time this will typically take.

When arriving in the aid station, let them know what you need for your feet. Advise them of any hot spots or blisters. Never let them pull shoes off your feet without proper unlacing. This action, however unintentional, can rupture a blister or cause increased pain to already hurting feet. A shoe horn can be a lifesaver to easily slide the heel out of and into the back of the shoe without too much pressure on sore and tender heels.

Part Three

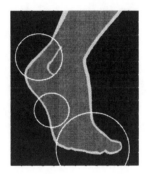

Treatments

21

Treatments to Fix Your Feet

"The 4th Law Of Running Injuries:
Virtually All Running Injuries Are Curable.
Only a minute fraction of true running injuries are not entirely
curable by quite simple techniques ..."
Tim Noakes, MD, *The Lore Of Running*.[16]

No matter how hard we try to prevent problems with our feet, there may come a time when repair is needed. Then you have to become reactive. This chapter explains how to fix foot problems that typically develop. It is always best to know how to fix problems before they develop. Beginning a long trail run or a multi-day hike without preparing for the possibility of blisters, a sprained ankle, or other potential injury is foolhardy. One or two unexpected blisters at the wrong time can spell the end to a long anticipated event.

Dave Covey, an experienced ultrarunner, in 1996 participated in a competitive and challenging 25-day 600 km wilderness trek across Western Australia which stressed his feet beyond his wildest imagination. While working in a walking and backpacking shoe store, he studied the different types of boots and selected a nylon and leather boot with a Gore-Tex fabric interior. The combination of high temperatures, long pants, and wearing heavy-duty nylon gaiters to protect his legs from the spiny vegetation made his legs sweat constantly. With his feet always wet, and the very uneven and rocky terrain, his feet were subject to extreme punishment.

Changing into dry wicking style socks every two hours helped for the first two days. By the third day blisters had developed on the bottoms of his toes. Moleskin simply would not adhere to the wet skin. By the end of the eighth day he rested his feet for a few days to try to dry out the blisters. He then used Betadine and duct tape on the toes. By the eighteenth day, the skin finally began to callous over and during the last six days of the trek he did not have to use any tape. Dave gave his boots high marks for comfort, realizing the blisters were caused by other factors.

When your feet are tired, there are several ways for you to help them feel better. When changing socks, stopping for lunch, or whenever possible, take a few minutes and massage your feet and check for any hot spots. A short soak in an icy stream or in a bucket of cold water can revitalize tired feet. When you sit down to change socks or shoes after being on your feet for any great length of time, elevating your feet above the level of your heart will help reduce swelling of the feet. While hiking or on adventure races, try to wash your feet with soap and water at least once per day, preferably in the evening.

The following chapters provide information on dealing with foot problems common to runners, hikers, and adventure racers. Included are descriptions of the problem, ways to treat the problem, products which can help relieve or solve the problem, and, in some cases, exercises to strengthen the afftected areas. Read the chapters that pertain to your injury history and try the treatments and products to find those that resolve your problems.

22

Hot Spots

Most runners experience hot spots in the areas where they are susceptible to blisters forming. The area will become sore and redness appears, thus the name "hot spot." There may also be a stinging or burning sensation. Around the reddened area will be a paler area which enlarges inward to where the skin is being rubbed.[17] The area becomes elevated as the surface skin is lifted as it fills with fluid. The hot spot has then become a blister.

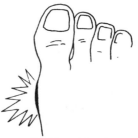

Reddened hot spot

We must deal with these hot spots before they become blisters. By the time the hot spot has developed enough to be felt, protection is necessary. Use your choice of one of the tapes or blister care products described in this book to protect the area. If you have used lubricants or powders on your feet, wipe the area with an alcohol wipe before applying tape, adhesive felt, or moleskin. Take the time to deal with hot spots as you feel them develop. Continuing to run or hike on them will only make them worse. They usually then turn into blisters which are harder to treat.

Examine your shoes or boots to determine whether you can modify them to remove the pressure point causing the problem. You may have to make a slit or cut out a small section in the side or toe of the shoe. Start with a small cut or hole and enlarge it as necessary.

23

Blisters

As all runners and hikers know, blisters can be painful. One blister, in a sensitive place on the foot, can easily ruin an otherwise good day. Blisters have often destroyed months of training and hundreds of dollars spent on a major event. Several blisters can reduce a runner to a walker or a hiker to a plodder, which in turn tends to create more blisters, which then slows forward motion even more. Too many of us fail to educate ourselves about blister prevention and how to do adequate blister care. Many runners and hikers think blisters are unavoidable and simply a part of the running or hiking process.

The time and conditions required for blisters to develop will vary from individual to individual. Runners and hikers tend to get either "downhill" blisters on the toes and forefoot caused by friction while going downhill and "uphill" blisters on the heels and over the Achilles tendons caused by friction while going uphill. Blisters on the heel can also mean the heel cup is too wide. Blisters on the top or front of the toes or the outsides of the outer toes can indicate friction in the toe box.

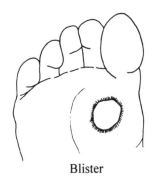

Blister

Blisters 101

A basic understanding of how blisters are formed is necessary in order to successfully treat them. Remember the triangle mentioned earlier (p.39)? The factors of heat, friction, and moisture around the triangle contribute to the formation of blisters. Studies have shown that the foot inside the shoe or boot is exposed to friction at many sites as it experiences motion from side to side, front to back, and up and down. These friction sites also change during the activity as the exercise intensity, movement of the sock, and flexibility of the shoe or boot changes.[18]

The outer epidermis layer of skin receives friction which causes it to rub against the inner dermis layer of skin. This friction between the layers of skin causes a blister to develop. As the outer layer of the epidermis is loosened from the deeper layers, the sac in between becomes filled with lymph fluid. A blister has then developed. If the blister is deep or traumatically stressed by continued running or hiking, the lymph fluid may contain blood. When the lymph fluid lifts the outer layer of epidermis, oxygen and nutrition to this layer is cut off and it becomes dead skin. This outer layer is easily burst. The fluid then drains and the skin loses its natural protective barrier. At this point the blister is most susceptible to infection.

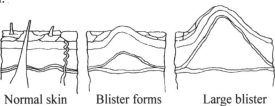

Normal skin   Blister forms   Large blister

The friction between the layers of skin is caused by the friction against whatever is touching the skin. As identified earlier, the majority of foot problems can be traced back to socks, powders, and lubricants — or the lack of them. In order to prevent blisters, friction must be reduced. Friction can be reduced in three main ways: 1) wearing double-layer socks or one inner and one outer sock, 2) keeping the feet dry by using powders, or 3) by using a lubricant to reduce chafing. It has been found that rubbing moist skin tends to produce higher friction than does rubbing skin that is either very dry or very wet.[19] Since the skin blisters more easily when soft and moist, it is important to understand the value of moisture-wicking socks coupled with knowing whether powders and/or lubricants are best for your feet and how to use them. Friction can also be reduced by eliminating pressure points caused by poor-fitting insoles and/or ill-fitting shoes. As stated earlier, examine your shoes or boots to try to eliminate the pressure point causing the blister. Cut slits or holes in the shoes as necessary.

Since blisters are caused by your footwear, the healing process truly begins when these are removed. If you have the option of a day's layover in camp without shoes and socks, this can speed the healing process and get you back on your feet faster and feeling better. Wearing sandals without socks exposes the blister to the air, which aids in healing.

Try to avoid getting blisters on top of existing blisters. When your skin is healing, protect or cushion the tender area.

Blisters Yesterday, Today, and Tomorrow

The problem which most of us face at one time or another is that what has worked for us in the past is no longer working. Ultrarunner Marv Skagerberg candidly warns "Caveat pedis, or let the toes beware. I have completely solved the blister problem 12 times by perfecting various methods which allow me to run for 24 hours and up, blister free. However the next time out with the exact same method, I have plenty of blisters." He has found that a combination of tincture of benzoin and silicone cream is by far the best for his feet. (See the section *Extreme Blister Prevention and Care* on page 114 for his method). Yesterday's method may have worked for years. Today's method may work for years. But then again, as Marv warns, it may not.

Tony Burke recalls the way he approached his 1996 back-pack of the 211 mile John Muir Trail in California's Sierra Nevada.

I had hoped that 15 years as a long distance runner and backpacker had eliminated the element of surprise in regards to foot problems and their treatment. I was wrong.

The first day of my 17 day hike required an additional 11 mile climb to the trailhead atop Mt. Whitney's 14,500 foot summit. On the way up, both heels started to blister. A little early in the trip I thought, but not unexpected. I immediately applied my favorite remedy, "2nd Skin." This was to become a daily ritual. The 2nd Skin would ease the soreness and keep the wounds reasonably clean but the Adhesive Knit that held it in place could not withstand the rigors of such a brutal, rocky trail and the blisters worsened to over an inch in diameter. Every step was painful, distracting me from the trail's beautiful surroundings. Soon, I ran out of Adhesive Knit, and resorted to that trusty standby, "duct tape." This kept the dressings in place longer, but, after clambering up and over yet another 12,000 foot pass, it too would slip. Then I got a rash from the tape's adhesive and smaller blisters from the tape's edges.

At my resupply point, nine days into the trip, I stocked up on 2nd Skin and duct tape, and padded the heel cups of my two-year old "broken-in" boots with moleskin and more duct tape. This stopped any future heel blistering but pushed my toes forward in the boots just enough to cause a whole new set of foot problems for the final leg of my trip. Some days it just isn't worth getting out of bed!

Tony's years of running and backpacking gave him a good base of experience — but he was venturing into new territory. The length of the trip, the rugged terrain, and the heavier backpack put added stresses on his feet.

The late ultrarunner Dick Collins used to have problems with blisters. After trying recommendations from others, including tape, he formed his own conclusion. Dick learned that for him, "... anything other than socks on his feet would over time become an irritant." He used only Vaseline on his feet and wore synthetic socks. Having completed 1037 races, including 238 ultras, he found what worked for him and stuck to it. Like Dick, we each need to learn what works for us and be open to trying new ideas and products that could help keep our feet healthy.

We have no guarantee that what works one day will work another day. Damon Lease experienced the frustration many athletes face when they do everything the same as they have done before and still blister. By mile 20 of a 50-mile race he was feeling hot spots on his toes. By mile 38 he was reduced to a painful walking state. At the 42.2 mile aid station he made the difficult decision to stop. Damon said, "I did nothing different in this race than any other ultra." He had used the same shoe and sock combination in other ultras but this course was steeper with "... more loose rocks and rough footing than the others." It happens. The trick is to play with all the variables in training to find what works best for your feet. Then be prepared with additional options in your gear bag.

General Blister Care

From the perspective of runners and hikers, the goal of blister treatments is to make the foot comfortable since often running or hiking must continue. Bryan P. Bergeron, MD., in an article "A Guide to Blister Management,"[20] identifies four therapeutic goals of blister management as: avoiding infection, minimizing pain and discomfort, stopping further blister enlargement, and maximizing recovery. He recommends all blister treatments be considered with these four goals in mind.

Avoiding infection

Stopping further blister enlargement

Four goals of blister management

Minimizing pain and discomfort

Maximizing recovery

For years, normal blister care has been gauze, moleskin, and Vaseline. Walking among the podiatrists at the finish line of a marathon or ultra, one finds most blister care practices incorporate these three materials.

The time-honored method of blister care uses moleskin to protect the blister. If the blister is intact, cut a piece of moleskin about 1/2" to 3/4" larger around than the blister, with a hole slightly larger than the blister in the center. Press it on the skin around the blister and put an antibiotic ointment, Bag Balm, or medicated Vaseline in the hole over the blister. The final step is to tape a piece of gauze over the moleskin. Adding a piece of adhesive knit or tape over the gauze will help hold it in place.

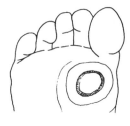

Moleskin with hole cut out for blister

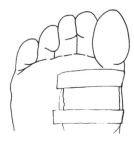

Gauze over moleskin

Alternatives to moleskin are adhesive felt, one of the tapes identified earlier, or Spenco Pressure Pads. You can also use one of the tapes or Spenco Skin Knit in place of the gauze.

If the above treatment does not help or if you must continue running or hiking, time should be taken to repair a blister before it enlarges and ruptures. Dr. Bergeron recommends draining the blister prior to applying a dressing when it is in a weight-bearing area and larger than 0.8" in diameter.[21] Use an alcohol wipe or hydrogen peroxide to clean the skin around the blister. Then use a pin or needle, flame-sterilized by heating with a match (avoid soot on the tip), to lance two to four puncture holes in a row in the blister. Making a single large hole increases the possibility of the blister roof shearing off when running or hiking must continue. Make the puncture holes on the side of the blister where ongoing foot pressure will push out additional fluid, generally to the back of the foot and towards the outside. Use pressure from your fingers to push out the fluid. Blot the fluid away with a tissue. Clean and dry the skin before doing further blister care. Apply a thin layer of antibiotic ointment at the puncture hole sites. The outer layer of dead skin should not be removed. It is important that the blister not be allowed to refill with fluid. Use one of the blister care products in the next section to protect the blister. Occasionally re-check the blister and drain it again if it has refilled with fluid.

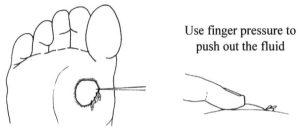

Use finger pressure to push out the fluid

Puncturing a blister with a needle

Do not drain a blister when it is blood-filled. To do so creates the risk of a serious infection as bacteria is easily introduced into the dermis layer of skin and into the blood system. Pad around the blister with moleskin or adhesive felt.

Do drain the blister if the fluid inside appears to be either cloudy or hazy. Normal blister fluid is clear and the change indicates that an infection has set in. The fluid needs to be drained, an antibiotic ointment applied, and a protective covering applied. Recheck the blister three times a day for signs of the infection returning. At that time, apply a new coating of antibiotic ointment and change the dressing. Early treatment can keep the infection from becoming more serious.

If the blister has ruptured, the degree of repair depends on the condition of the blister's outer covering. A simple ruptured blister where the skin is generally intact can be treated by a layer of antibiotic ointment over the blister and one of the blister care methods described in the next section.

If the outer layer of skin is torn off or only a flap of skin is left, carefully cut off the loose skin, clean the area and cover the new skin with an antibiotic ointment. Then use one of the blister care methods described in the next section. Valerie Doyle uses a hair dryer on the blister when the outer layer of skin has been removed or torn off. She has found the low heat and drying action speeds the healing process.

Blisters should be rechecked daily for signs of infection. An infected blister may be both seen and felt. An infection will be indicated by any of the following: redness, swelling, red streaks up the limb, pain, fever, and pus. The blister must be treated as a wound. It must be frequently cleaned and an antibiotic ointment applied. Frequent warm water or Epson Salt soaks can also help the healing process. Stay off the foot as much as possible and elevate it above the level of your heart. If the infection does not seem to subside over 24 to 48 hours, see a doctor.

The use of an antibiotic ointment for open blisters is important to avoid infection. While you may not put an ointment on an open blister while in the middle of a run or the middle of the day while backpacking, at the end of the event or day, take the necessary time to properly treat the open skin. Check your local drug store for a broad spectrum antibiotic ointment like Neosporin® or Polysporin® which provides protection against both gram-positive and gram-negative pathogens.

Adhesive Felt   Adhesive felt is available in rolls in 1/8″ and 1/4″ thicknesses. This pink felt is extra thick, and compared to moleskin, provides extra cushioning and a stronger adhesive base. Check with your local drug store, medical supply store, or podiatrist for its availability. Hapad, Inc. is a mail-order source for adhesive surgical felt made from a rayon and wool blend in a roll 1/4″ thick by 6″ by 7.5 feet.

Moleskin   Moleskin is a soft, cotton padding which protects skin surfaces against friction and has an adhesive backing which adheres to the skin. Dr. Scholl's® makes Moleskin Plus from thin cotton flannel padding and Moleskin Foam from soft latex foam. Moleskin is available in most drug stores, in a variety of sizes and can be cut-to-size. Hapad, Inc. is a mail order source for moleskin in a roll 1/8″ thick by 6″ by 7.5 feet. Moleskin should not be applied directly over a blister because it can tear any loose blister skin when removed.

Spenco Pressure Pads   Spenco Pressure Pads are made from closed-cell polyethylene foam which is soft, flexible and thin. It is available in a six-pack of 3″ by 5″ sheets with two pre-cut pads with ovals and circles and two uncut pads to be used over hot spots and blisters.

Advanced Blister Care

Even though the time-honored blister care products are still used by many, there are more efficient products to both prevent blisters and promote healing.

The chapter *Taping for Blisters* contains much information which can be used as treatments for blisters. See the sections *Taping Basics* on page 67, *Duct Tape Techniques* on page 70, and *Suzi T's Taping Technique* on page 72 for a complete description on how to use taping as a treatment. By following the methods described, tape can be applied over a blister, whether the blister roof is intact or not. Tape can also be applied over Spenco 2nd Skin or other blister care products mentioned below.

Tincture of benzoin applied to the area around a hot spot or blister will help blister products or tapes stick to the skin more effectively. Avoid getting tincture into a broken blister or other broken skin. After the tincture has dried, apply one of the blister care products below. Be sure to apply a light coating of powder or lubricant to counteract the still exposed tincture of benzoin to prevent socks or contaminants from sticking to the skin. Be forewarned that forgetting this step when using tincture of benzoin on the toes may result in blisters from two toes being stuck together.

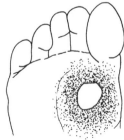
Tincture of benzion applied
around blister

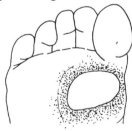
Blister product placed over
blister

When using any of the products listed below on your blisters, be sure to occasionally check them. They may peel off, shift their position, or ball up under the stresses of hiking and running. When doing hills, the constant uphill and downhill movements of the feet combined with the pressures of the running body or the weight of a backpack may compromise their integrity. If you sense a change in how they feel, stop and check it out.

Compeed®   Compeed is a blister covering made with an elastic polyurethane film over a moisture absorbing and adhering layer, both covered with protective silicone papers which are removed for use. Functioning like a second layer of skin, Compeed cushions the area, virtually eliminating blister pain, while protecting it from further damage caused by friction. Tapered edges help adherence to the skin without rolling. It is meant to be used *without being cut* and can be worn for several days. For larger blisters, put two pieces side-by-side. Be careful not to wrinkle the edges of the pads.

Compeed's hydrocolloid construction creates optimum conditions for rapid healing while embedded cellulose particles absorb excess fluid and perspiration from the wound surfaces. Additionally, bacteria is sealed out, reducing the risk of infection.

Long-distance hiker and ultrarunner Brick Robbins uses tincture of benzoin around his blisters and then applies a Compeed pad. The pad usually will stay on for three to five days before falling off. After dealing with massive blisters, Steve Benjamin learned to use a Compeed pad placed over each spot prone to blistering, overlapping them where necessary. He then puts tape over the Compeed pads to hold them in place. Using five pads per foot, he has eliminated his blister problem. This type of trial can be done with any blister prevention products.

Compeed comes in two sizes, a 3.5″ by 1″ strip and a 2.75″ by 1.75″ oval, which are available in plastic compacts with five pieces inside. Look for Compeed at drug, running, and sports stores. For more information contact Bruder Healthcare Company.

Mueller's More Skin   Mueller's More Skin pads have the feel and consistency of human skin, removing friction between two moving surfaces. More Skin is available in 3″ circles,

1″ circles and squares, and 3″ squares. Available only by wholesale purchase. For more information contact Mueller Sports Medicine.

Spenco 2nd Skin® Dressings　　2nd Skin Dressings are a unique skin-like hydrogel pad which can be applied directly over closed or open blisters. The pads help reduce friction and the discomfort of blisters. They can also be used over abrasions, cuts, or similar wounds. Use one or more pads to cover the blister area. Remove the cellophane layer on one side of the pad, apply that gel side to the blister, and then remove the cellophane from the other side. The pads do not stick to the skin, requiring tape to hold them on the skin. They should be kept moist and changed daily. Cover the 2nd Skin pads with either Spenco Adhesive Knit, one of the tapes mentioned, or moleskin. These pads are available in a variety of sizes: 1″ squares, 3″ circles, and 3″ by 4″ and 3″ by 6.5″ rectangles. Some sizes are non-sterile while others are sold as sterile Moist Burn Pads. Be sure to keep your packet of pads moist or they will dry out.

Spenco® Adhesive Knit　　Use Spenco Adhesive Knit to cover 2nd Skin pads or as a skin protector to prevent blisters. Spenco Adhesive Knit is a highly breathable woven fiber with the ability to stretch and conform and does not sweat or bathe off. It cuts to size, fitting easily around toes and hard to tape areas. Adhesive Knit comes in 3″ by 5″ rectangles in a six-pack.

Spyroflex®　　Spyroflex, made by PolyMedica Healthcare, Inc., is an adhesive sterile wound dressing. It consists of a thin two-layered polyurethane membrane that has an adhesive inner side which goes against the skin and an outer layer which is moisture-vapor-permeable and microporous. As an "intelligent" dressing, Syproflex is open-cell constructed for moisture management that helps protect the blister from external moisture and bacteria while speeding the healing process. Moisture from the blister is absorbed by the porous membrane, passes through, and evaporates. The membrane is water resistant, not allowing water to pass through to the blister. The pad, cut to size, is applied directly over the blister and may be left on for up to seven days, yet is easily removed without sticking or tearing. Spyroflex works extremely well on inflamed and infected blisters. For maximum adherence, use as much of the pad as possible on the skin around the blister and cover the pad with Spenco Adhesive Knit or a similar porous tape. If continuing to run or hike, check the pad occasionally to be sure it remains in place.

Spyroflex is available in an Abrasion Dressing Kit with three 4″ square pads, a Blister Dressing Kit with five 2″ square pads, and a Skin Savers package with eight pads in the two different sizes. All pads may be cut to size. They are applied directly over the blister, are water resistant, and may be removed without sticking. For more information contact PolyMedica Healthcare, Inc.

Coban™ Carry a roll of 3M's 2″ Coban in your blister repair kit. Coban is a self-adherent wrap which can be used around feet, ankles, and heels to hold blister products in place. Its elasticity and flexibility allows movement of the joints. Since it adheres to itself, it contains no adhesive. Because it is elastic, be careful not to apply it too tight and cause constriction. Your pharmacy or medical supply store typically carry Coban or similar self-adherent wraps. Most are available in 2″, 3″, and 4″ widths.

Extreme Blister Prevention and Care

There are athletes who may choose to use extreme methods to initially prevent blisters or subsequently treat their blisters in order to continue on in a competitive event. These are aggressive methods. A competitive 100-mile, 24-hour, 48-hour, or six-day run may cause a runner to want to try any means to keep running. Likewise, hikers may need to deal aggressively with blisters when in the middle of a multi-day hike. The team participation rule in an adventure racing event may force a team member to consider treating blisters in an extreme method.

There are several extreme methods for extreme blister prevention and care. Review the following methods to determine whether one may be useful for you in your running and hiking adventures.

The first extreme method simply uses information from the chapter *Taping for Blisters* which can be used as an aggressive treatment for both blister prevention and treatment. See the sections *Taping Basics* on page 67, *Duct Tape Techniques* on page 70, and

Suzi T's Taping Technique on page 72 for a complete description on how to tape. By following the methods described, tape can be applied over a blister, whether the blister roof is intact or not.

The second extreme method of blister prevention uses tincture of benzoin, or a similar benzoin based product, and silicone cream. Marv Skagerberg still likes his benzoin and silicone cream combination which worked for him for the last 78 of 86 days of the 1985 cross-country Trans America race. Averaging 43 miles per day through 12 states, Marv did not get a single blister with this method.

1. Clean the feet thoroughly and dry completely.
2. Coat the feet, heels, soles, and toes with tincture of benzoin.
3. Let the feet dry for three minutes, keeping the toes spread. The feet will still be quite sticky.
4. Apply a silicone cream. He uses Avon's Silicone Glove which comes in a 1.5 ounce tube and is available through your Avon sales representative.
5. Put on a lightweight double-layer sock.
6. Reapply the cream every four to six hours and change socks at the same time.

Bill Trolan, MD, uses C & M Pharmacal's Hydropel Protective Silicone Ointment over Cramer's Tuf Skin in the same manner as Marvin described above. He recommends reapplying the benzoin product and cream at every sock change.

Dr. Trolan has participated in several Raid Gaulloises and served as a medical consultant to adventure racing teams in the Eco-Challenge as well as to Naval Special Warfare. He wrote the *Blister Fighter Guide*,[22] which is included in the Blister Fighter Medical Kit available through Outdoor Research. He describes two more extreme methods of treating blisters, warning that they are "... not for the faint of heart." This treatment method has helped many adventure racers finish their events. The methods are *not* to be used if the blister is infected. After the blister is opened and drained thoroughly and the feet are dried, use one of the following methods to seal down the blister roof.

☞ Use a syringe, without a needle, to inject tincture of benzoin directly into the blister. Immediately apply pressure across the top of the blister to evenly seal down the blister's outer layer to the underlying skin. This also pushes out any extra benzoin. Be forewarned that injecting the benzoin is momentarily painful. Dr. Trolan rates it as an eight on a one to ten pain scale where "... childbirth and kidney stones are a ten and a paper cut is a one."

☞ Use New Skin Liquid Bandage, instead of benzoin, injected into the blister. This does not seal the blister either as well or as long as benzoin but is less painful. He rates it as a five or six on the pain scale. See page 64 for information on New Skin Liquid Bandage.

At the 1996 Western States 100 Mile Endurance Run Teresa Krall found out the hard way how painful tincture in a blister can be. The cotton ball used to apply the tincture was dropped into the dirt and one of her crew mistakenly decided to pour the tincture directly onto her blistered heel. As Brick Robbins, her pacer, recalls, "The tincture of benzoin was poured before I could object, followed by a blood curdling scream. After a while (it seemed like forever), Teresa quit screaming." Teresa recalls the blister being about half dollar size and the pain being intense. She would not do it again unless it was the only method left to let her run, but would try Compeed first. George Freelen, a former Army Ranger, recalls when he was in the Army he used the tincture to seal blisters. He vividly remembers, "It hurts like hell, but only for 15 to 20 seconds." The choice is yours. It works to seal the blister's roof to the inner skin so running and hiking can continue. But there is definitely pain and always the risk of infection.

After sealing the blister, Dr. Trolan gives several options. Apply a coating of tincture of benzoin to help the tape or moleskin better adhere to the skin. Or you may apply Instant Krazy® Glue over the blister. This layer provides an extra layer of protection and helps your tape covering better adhere to the skin. Do not use Krazy Glue in the blister.

For severe cases, Dr. Trolan has used the tincture of benzoin injection, followed by a coating of tincture of benzoin on top of the blister, followed by a coating of New Skin Liquid Bandage, followed by a layer of Krazy Glue, and finally followed by tape or moleskin. He recommends using an emery board or fine nail file to smooth any rough spots on the blister coating before applying tape or moleskin.

When using tape or moleskin over a blister, apply it as smoothly as possible. Use finger pressure to smooth it evenly across the blister and then repeat the smoothing process several more times after the initial application. Remember to cut the tape or moleskin large enough to extend well beyond the edges of the blister. The most common failure in using tape or moleskin is not allowing enough necessary for good adherence. The larger the blister, the more the tape or moleskin should extend past its edges.

When using moleskin over blisters, he recommends using a razor to shave the moleskin, after it is applied, to remove its tiny fibers. The fibers can later catch on socks which exerts pull against the blister.

Dr. Trolan suggests caution in using the two extreme methods described above. Possible permanent damage to the skin surfaces is possible. Use these methods only if you are willing to accept the possible consequences.

While you may see medical aid station people using syringes with needles to draw out the blister fluid and then to inject the tincture, an explanation is necessary. Syringes with needles must be sterile in order to prevent infection. There is no safe way to dispose of the syringes and needles, or "sharps" as they are called in the medical profession, except in a sharps container. In the outdoors this presents a problem. Syringes and needles should never be used on more than one person. In this day of hepatitis and AIDS, we need to practice universal precautions: in this case gloves and hand washing before each person being worked on. An open blister must be treated as an open wound and the blister's fluid must be treated as a bodily fluid. Additionally, there are two more concerns. With a syringe you might inject more tincture than is necessary to get a good seal or not enough to cover all inner surfaces. By making several small puncture holes in the blister, and using a syringe without a needle, excess tincture can be pushed out when pressure is applied to the roof of the blister. A good seal is then ensured.

Beyond Blisters

There may be times when blisters develop and even with treatment, due to continued running or hiking, additional care is needed. Several things may happen. The skin may slough off and ball up in the sock, leaving raw exposed skin. The skin may stay in place, but fall off when the sock is removed. The raw skin may bleed. When blisters have developed to this point, a choice will have to be made. Continuing to run or hike may lead to infection. Ideally, stay off the feet as much as possible. If you must continue, treat the problem and recheck the dressing frequently.

Sterile wound dressing products will help the healing process:

☞ PolyMedica Healthcare's Spyroflex (4″ x 4″ adhesive polyure-thane membrane)

☞ Spenco's 2nd Skin Moist Burn Pads (1.5″ x 2″, 2″ x 3″, and 3″ x 4″ thin gel sheets)

☞ Cramer Products' Nova Derm™ (4″ x 4″ and 3″ x 6″ glycerine gel formula)

☞ Mueller Sports Medicine's Dermal Pads (4″ x 4″ closed cell elastomer)

☞ Bristol-Meyers Squibb's DuoDERM® and DuoDERM® Extra Thin (4″ x 4″ and 8″ x 8″)

Use these products over the blister or raw skin and leave them on as the healing process begins from the inside. The non-adhesive dressings require a Coban or gauze wrap to hold them in place. These dressings are typically available only through medical supply stores. One of these carried on a multi-day hike could easily save one's feet. Race directors should consider having several in their first-aid kit.

Fixing Blisters, Their Way or Your Way

Dr. Trolan stresses the importance of understanding how your feet change when you add things to them. Adding moleskin and gauze to your foot changes the way your foot fits inside your shoe or boot. The extra thickness of the blister patch changes pressures and angles of the foot inside the shoe. This in turn changes the shoe from its usually "broken-in" fit to that of a "mismatch." New pressure points develop, turning first into new hot spots and then into blisters. The biomechanics of the foot and ankle and leg are altered and the gait changes. Additional problems are likely to develop. Dr. Trolan recommends using as little and as thin a blister patch as possible.

This becomes most important when participating in an event where you do not have control over the blister treatments and how they are applied. Participate in a 100-mile trail event or an Eco-Challenge and you will find medical aid stations manned by podiatrists, podiatry students, nurses, emergency medical technicans, and an assortment of individuals with various medical skills. These individuals will treat your blisters according to what they know and what materials they have available to them. How they treat your blisters may not be how you would like them treated. Most aid stations are stocked with moleskin, Vaseline, and gauze. They may or may not have 2nd Skin, alcohol wipes, and tincture of benzoin. If you want your feet treated with Compeed, Spyroflex, or another product, you will have to carry a few pieces of these in your fanny pack. If you want a specific powder or lubricant you will need to carry these in a small container.

Do not hesitate to give medical personnel at these aid stations instruction on how you would like your feet patched. I remember the bulky gauze patch put on the bottom of my right foot in 1986 during the final stages of my first Western States 100 Mile Endurance Run. While it was a good patch job, it simply did not fit right and turned me from a runner into a walker. Be aware of how they are treating your feet. It is up to you to advise them of any special methods of blister patching you want them to use on your feet.

24

Stubbed Toes, Bruises, Sprains, and Strains

Occasionally we stub our toes resulting in a hematoma, a bruise, or a fracture. Ankle sprains and strains are also common occurrences. The cause may be rocks or tree roots hidden in leaves or grasses, trail running at night, or twisting motions coming off a curb.

Stubbed toes are more common in running shoes than in hiking boots. Stubbing a toe on a rock or tree root can be very painful. Check the toe for discoloration which can indicate a deep bruise or a fracture. Treatment includes "buddy taping," icing the toe (a cold stream will also work), elevation, and a firm soled shoe or boot. Buddy taping is done by lightly taping the injured toe to the toe next to it, with a piece of cotton between (never tape skin-to-skin). For elevation to be effective, the injured toe should be above the level of the heart. If the injury does not respond to treatment, medical treatment and an X-ray may be necessary.

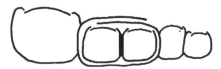

With cotton between toes, lightly tape
the injured toe to a good toe

Ankles are frequently sprained or strained. A sprain is a stretching or tearing injury to the ligaments that stabilize bones together at a joint. You may experience sudden pain or hear a pop.

After a sprain the fibrous joint capsule swells and becomes inflamed, discolored, and painful. A strain is a stretching or tearing injury to a muscle or its tendon that attaches the muscle to the bone. There may be bleeding into the muscle area which can cause swelling, pain, stiffness, and muscle spasm followed by a bruise.

Since ligaments and tendons do not have their own direct blood supply, their healing is slow. Karl King found that the nutritional supplements of one gram Glycine, one gram Lysine, and one-half gram buffered Vitamin C, and one Aleve® tablet is helpful in the healing process. Take this combination at breakfast and at bedtime. The supplements provide the major building blocks for connective tissue while the Aleve is an anti-inflammatory.

The most common ankle sprain is an "inversion" sprain where the foot rolls to the outside and the ankle turns out. The injured area is just below the ankle joint on the outside of the foot. Rapid swelling and discoloration occurs. Less common is the "eversion" sprain where the ankle is turned inward. An X-ray will reveal whether there is a bone fracture which would require immobilization of the joint.

The treatment for a sprain or strain includes the classic RICE treatment, where R = rest, I = ice, C = compression, and E = elevation. The first 24 hours are the most critical for beginning treatment.

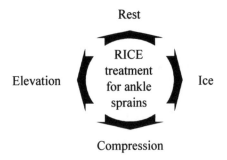

Early treatment decreases swelling and lessens the risk of additional injury. Initial rest of the foot is also important. A lightly wrapped Ace® wrap will provide compression to help keep swelling down while providing support. Apply the Ace wrap from the forefoot towards the ankle. Do not wear the Ace wrap at night. Apply ice for 20 minutes at a time at least four times daily. Do not place ice directly on the skin. Always use a thin towel, washcloth, or T-shirt between the ice bag and the skin. When at home, a bag of frozen peas or corn works nicely to conform to the ankle curves. Avoid icing for more than 20 minutes at a time. The injured area should be elevated above the level of the heart as much as possible during the first 48 hours. The treatment goal is to return the ankle to normal motion and to be weight-bearing as soon as possible. The use of anti-inflammatory medications is usually warranted.

Ice massage to reduce swelling can be done by freezing water in a paper or foam cup. When frozen, remove part of the cup and rub the ice around the injured area. Because it cools the area faster than normal icing, limit the massage to six to eight minutes.

Heat increases blood flow to an injured area, which makes swelling worse. For this reason, the use of heat is not recommended for at least a week after an injury. Moist heat can be applied by using a moist heating pad, a warm towel, or a warm bath. Dry heat can be applied by using a heating pad for 20 minutes at a time.

Strengthening exercises for the foot and ankle can help prevent injuries in the first place and then help in recovery from an injury. Writing the alphabet with your toes simulates ankle motion in all directions. Moving the ankle up and down in a pumping motion helps decrease swelling. Isometric exercises with the feet pushing against each other helps strengthen muscles without joint movement. Push down with the foot on top while pulling up with the foot on the bottom. Then reverse feet. You can also put your feet bottom-to-bottom, first pushing the big toes against each other and then the small toes against each other. Hold the motions for six to ten seconds and repeat several times a day.

Mike Bate found he could eliminate ankle problems by doing a simple exercise. He recommends strengthening ankles by balancing with one foot flat on the ground and the other leg bent back at the knee, as if you were in the normal support phase of a running stride. Practice until you can hold your balance for four to five minutes. When you have mastered this step, close your eyes and do the same thing. Without eye feedback, it is harder to maintain your balance. Repeatedly losing your balance and then recovering gradually strengthens the ankles even more.

Delayed treatments for sprains or strains increases the risk of swelling and further injury.

Ankle Supports

Weak ankles can be a problem, particularly on trails. After a turned or sprained ankle, an ankle support will often provide the support and protection necessary for light training. Weak ankles can also benefit from an ankle support. Adhesive taping of the ankle can be helpful, however, for it to be effective someone who is experienced must do the taping. While taping restricts extreme motion, the tape loses strength as it moves with the skin. Forty percent of its strength can be lost within 20 minutes.

Ankle supports are typically made from a compression type sock. Some offer a figure-8 style stretch wrap which gives additional strength and support. Since the supports vary in fit and material, experiment wearing the support against the skin or over a sock to find the best fit on your foot. All the ankle supports listed below are compact in size and fit easily into a fannypack or back-pack. If you are prone to ankle injuries, consider carrying one as a preventative measure.

Cho-Pat® Ankle Support   The Cho-Pat Ankle Support provides compression to the ankle with a removable Velcro fastener which wraps in a figure-8 around the ankle giving additional compression at specific locations of the ankle while providing stabilization. The support is made of neoprene. The unisex sizes are based on body weight. It is available by mail order from Cho-Pat, Inc.

Cropper Medical Bio Skin™   Cropper Medical makes a superb product called Bio Skin. The Bio Skin is made up of a Lycra knit outer layer, a SmartSkin™ membrane which absorbs moisture and wicks it from the skin, a Lycra knit/fleece inner layer, and a SkinLok™ layer against the skin. Bio Skin stretches with the body's movement while giving compression without bunching and binding and does not constrict the joints. The SmartSkin membrane provides higher levels of moisture vapor transmission as the activity produces more perspiration and heat. The three designs include a standard ankle skin, a figure-8 ankle skin, and visco ankle skin with a figure-8 wrap. The Bio Skin material will not tear even if cut into. Cropper Medical also makes models for knee problems or injuries, including hinged braces for runners needing knee support. For more information contact Cropper Medical.

Kallassy Ankle Support®   The Kallassy Ankle Support is a proven design for rehabilitation of severe ankle sprains. The support is made of nylon-lined neoprene that provides warmth and compression. Stability is provided first by a strap that wraps around the ankle and secondly by a non-stretch lateral strapping system that helps prevent inversion motions of the ankle. If you are prone to turned ankles, this support is one of the most stabilizing ankle supports offered. A lace-up version is offered but it would not be as comfortable for running and hiking. The Kallassy is offered by the Rebound Orthopedic Supports Division of Tecnol. For more information contact Tecnol Consumer Products.

Perform 8™ Lateral Ankle Stabilizer   The Perform 8 provides excellent external stabilization of the ankle's lateral (outer) ligaments, similar to ankle taping. While a lightweight elastic compression stocking provides support to soft tissue, an elastic figure-8 configuration strap wraps around the foot. Pads relieve pressure on the Achilles tendon. For more information contact Brown Medical Industries.

Stromgren Supports Inc.   A good ankle support is made by Stromgren Supports Inc. Their double strap model offers a unique sock style support with two elastic straps which wrap around the ankle to provide the benefit of taped ankle support without the tape. This product has a fairly loose fit and folded-over sewn edges at the forefoot and the heel cutout which may provide irritation on long runs. For more information contact Stromgren Supports Inc.

Additional ankle supports can usually be found in drug stores and sporting goods stores. Three examples are those made by Cramer, Mueller, and Spenco. Cramer's neoprene ankle support wraps around the ankle. Mueller's Neoprene Ankle Support is a one-piece support with stretch nylon on each side. The Spenco Fiberflex™ is an elastic bandage for the ankle made from elastic and transverse nylon fibers. Ace wraps, or similar style roll-wraps are helpful after a sprain, but provide little support against initially turning your ankle.

25

Toenail Problems

Runners and hikers need to maintain good toenail care. Toenails should be trimmed regularly, straight across the nail — never rounded at the corners. After trimming toenails, use a nail file to smooth the top of the nail down toward the front of the toe and remove any rough edges. If you draw your finger from the skin in front of the toe up across the nail and can feel a rough edge, the nail can be trimmed shorter or filed smoother.

Ingrown toenails, most common to the big toe, may cause infection and require medical attention. Soak your foot in warm water or Epson Salts two to three times a day to reduce the infection. If you cannot trim the nail yourself, check with your orthopedist or podiatrist.

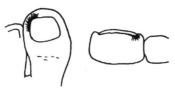

Ingrown toenail, most common on the big toe

Fungus under and around the nails should be treated promptly with antifungal medications. See the chapter *Athlete's Foot* on page 149 for information on treating fungal infections.

The technical name for the runner's black toenail, "subungal hematoma," is simply a blood-filled swelling under the nail. This common occurrence is caused by the trauma of the toe or toes repetitively bumping against the front of the shoe. Individuals with Morton's foot are most susceptible to having black toenails. The nail becomes discolored and usually has associated pain. To relieve pressure from a black toenail, use one of the following methods depending on the look of the toenail. The treatment may have to be repeated several times. Although the two methods below might sound painful, they are usually not painful.

1. If the discoloration does not extend to the end of the toenail, swab the nail with an alcohol wipe, and use a match to heat a pin, needle, or in a pinch, a paper clip, and gently penetrate the nail with the heated point. The blood will ooze through the hole. Keep slight pressure on the nail bed to help expel the built-up blood. Stopping too soon will cause the blood to clot in the hole and the problem will reoccur.

2. If the discoloration extends to the end of the toenail, use a sterile pin or needle to penetrate the skin under the nail and release the pressure. Holding slight pressure on the nailbed will help expel the blood.

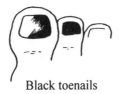

Black toenails

Care must be taken to prevent a secondary bacterial infection through the hole in the nail or at the end of the nail by using an antibiotic ointment and covering the site with a Band-Aid®. Loss of the nail usually follows in the months ahead. The new nail will begin growing, pushing up the old nail and may come in looking odd. Do not be concerned about the process unless an infection develops. Dr. David Hannaford, a podiatrist, tells of patients who come to see him thinking they "... have cancer" because their nails are growing in funny-looking.

Many runners are simply prone to black toenails. Some runners choose to have them surgically removed. The best means of preventing black toenails is to wear shoes with a generous toe box and the proper length for your feet. Paul Vorwerk used to think shoes should fit tight "... like a surgeon's glove," but after losing nails on his big toes, he now runs in shoes with good toe space. Some runners cut slits in their shoe's toe box or cut out a portion of the toe box to gain relief. You may find relief by wearing a metatarsal pad, a small circular pad that pushes up the ball of the foot and drops the toes down, which takes pressure off the toenails. Contact Hapad, Inc. for information on these pads.

If you stub your toe and the nail is bent backwards, the key is to prevent the toenail from catching on your sock and tearing off. Wrap either a Band-Aid or tape around the toe to hold the toenail in place. The use of an antibiotic ointment under the nail will help prevent infection.

26

Morton's Foot

Morton's foot is a common problem where second toe (next to the big toe) is longer than the big toe. The repeated pressure of the longer second toe against the front of the shoe or boot may traumatize the nail. If a hemotoma develops under the nail, the nail will change color and may fall off.

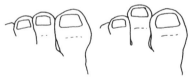

Morton's foot is when the first
toe is longer than the big toe

To get a good fit, look for shoes or boots with a wide toe box. It may be necessary to use a shoe or boot one or more sizes larger than normal in order to have space for the longer first toe. The use of a non-slippery insole will keep the foot from sliding forward. Look for an insole with a good heel cup, an arch that fits your foot, and a surface material which grips the foot and sock. Some runners will cut a slit over or on either side of the toe to relieve pressure. Another option is to cut out a small piece of the toe box over the toe. Orthotics may also provide relief.

27

Heel Problems

The most common cause of heel pain is incorrect movement of the foot during running, hiking, or walking. Heel pain may be caused by heel spurs or plantar fasciitis as the heel bone and attached soft tissues are stressed. Heel spurs are small points of bone sticking out from the "calcaneus" heel bone. Stresses to the plantar fascia where it inserts into the calcaneus cause heel spurs to develop. A heel spur can usually be seen on a X-ray. A heel bruise or stone bruise is pain felt directly under the calcaneus. This pain is usually tenderness at a small site in the heel pad on the bottom of the heel. As we age, the thickness of this heel pad decreases and our natural shock absorption is reduced, making us more susceptible to injury.

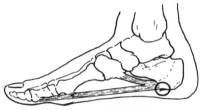

Heel spur at the bottom
of the heel bone

Heel pads and cups may help heel spurs, plantar fasciitis, calcaneal bursitis, heel and arch discomfort, heel neuromas, and nerve entrapment syndromes. Proper conditioning of the feet and gradually working up to longer distances can help minimize heel pain. Resting your feet and using ice is helpful when you first experience pain — for 20 minutes three to four times a day for several days. Later, warm soaks can help. If the problem persists, make an appointment with a podiatrist or orthopedist.

Stretching can help resolve heel pain. Slowly stretch the toes upwards towards the head at least three times per day, holding the stretch for at least 15 seconds. Do this stretching in the morning before getting out of bed. Warm soaks and stretching after extended sitting can also be beneficial.

A study by the American Orthopaedic Foot and Ankle Society looked at heel pain related to plantar fasciitis.[23] Dr. Glenn Pfeffer reported chronic heel pain as the most common foot problem with up to 80% caused by proximal plantar fasciitis. The study compared a common polypropylene custom orthotic device, three over-the-counter heel pads, and stretching alone. After comparing the results of five control groups, they found that stretching and over-the-counter heel pads were as effective as stretching and the more costly orthotics. Their recommendation is "... for the initial treatment of heel pain, stretching, and a simple, inexpensive, off-the-counter device is the best way to go."

The heel cups and pads listed below are quite varied. Some heel cups have a waffle design on the bottom of the cup, others have a special-density bottom material. Most heel cups simply cup the heel while others are incorporated into a sock design. Heel pads are small and fit easily into a shoe to provide cushioning. Try several to find a design that works best for your pain or injury. Heel cups and pads are small and can easily be carried as a preventative measure if you are prone to heel pain. The PSC wrap is a small alternative to heel cups and pads. Several off-the-counter orthotics are also available.

Cramer Heel Cup　　　　Cramer Products offers a basic heel cup made with Provosane II™ bonded to soft polyurethane foam. For more information contact Cramer Products Inc.

Hapad Heel Pads and Cushions　　　　Hapad's Heel Cushions are useful in treating heel pain associated with stone bruises, heel spurs, leg length discrepancies, and Achilles tendinitis. The Horseshoe Heel Pads relieve heel pain and the Medial/Lateral

Heel Wedges help correct misalignment of the heel and ankle. The Comf-Orthotic 3/4-Length Insole is a contoured one-piece arch, metatarsal, and heel cushion which relieves heel spur pain. The coiled, spring-like wool fibers provide firm and resilient support as they mold and shape to the foot. For more information contact Hapad, Inc.

Heel Bed 4pf   UCO International makes a Heel Bed 4pf, a molded polymer orthotic device for the relief of heel pain secondary to plantar fasciitis. Its molded design cups the heel and has an arch support. These are made in sizes small, medium, and large. This heel bed has to be ordered through a distributor, a podiatrist, or a orthopedist.

Heel Hugger™   The Heel Hugger is designed to treat heel pain and inflammatory problems of the heel. The neoprene sock design surrounds the heel to the mid-foot providing support, stabilization, and compression to control edema. Gel pads with Sealed Ice™ provide additional stabilization and cold therapy on either side of the calcaneus heel bone. The Heel Hugger provides relief from spurs, plantar fasciitis, Achilles tendinitis, heel contusions, narrow heels, and rearfoot instability. For more information contact Brown Medical Industries.

Lynco Biomechanical Orthotic Systems   Apex offers the Lynco Biomechanical Orthotic System, a "ready-made" triple-density orthotic system that comes in enough variations to accommodate 90% of foot disorders, including pain from heel spurs and heel pain syndrome. See the chapter *Orthotics* on page 77 for more information on these orthotics.

PSC™ by fabrifoam   The PSC is a pronation/spring control device. It is designed to treat chronic heel pain, heel spur syndrome, plantar fasciitis, and shin splints. This reusable strapping device is made from a lightweight, thin foam elastic which breaths and is easily placed on the foot. It wraps under the arch to provide support to the plantar fascia and then around the heel to reduce the force of heel strike and biomechanically move the foot's mid-line to a more neutral position. For more information contact fabrifoam Products.

Spur Relief Heel Cup   Orthopedic Product Sales makes a Spur Relief Heel Cup with silicone that has a density similar to that of human tissue. For more information contact Orthopedic Product Sales.

Tuli's Heel Cups   Tuli's makes heel cups for runners and hikers. The TuliGel Heel Cup offers a double-ribbed waffle design with gel polymer which is soft but strong. Their Tuli's® Pro Heel Cup™ has a double-ribbed waffle design while the Standard Heel Cup™ is made with a single waffle design. For more information contact Allor Medical, Inc.

Some runners and hikers may find relief using a basic heel cushion, a simple pad which fits under the heel of the foot. Spenco and Spectrum Sports offer heel cushions. Check your running, backpacking, or drug stores for these and similar products.

28

Plantar Fasciitis

The plantar fascia is a band of connective fibrous tissue that runs from the heel to the ball of the foot, forming the foot's arch. The band aids in support and stabilization of the foot during hiking and running. The arch flattens when standing. As you begin a step the heel lifts up and the plantar fascia tightens to form the curve of the arch and provides a strong push off with the toes. An inflammation of the fascia, called plantar fasciitis, most often occurs with overuse. The stretching and tearing of some of the fibers in the plantar fascia as it inserts into the heel bone causes the inflammation. If you have flat feet or if you over-pronate, the plantar fascia is strained, mainly at the heel. The stresses of running and hiking may flatten, lengthen, and eventually cause small tears in the plantar fascia. Tears near the heel bone may cause a heel spur to develop.

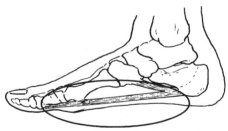

Plantar fascia

Plantar fascia pain is commonly felt in the morning or after long periods of sitting. The first steps at these times causes a sudden strain to the band of tissue. There may be either heel or arch pain. The pain and stiffness is usually centered at the bottom of the heel, but symptoms may radiate into the arch. Although the pain may decrease somewhat with your initial activity, as the day progresses, it may return and be quite painful.

Treatments include moist heat and stretching in the morning or before activity, icing massage after activity, changing insoles or adding an arch support, taping of the foot or an arch brace, foot exercises, and shoe modifications. In extreme cases oral anti-inflammatory medications, cortisone injections, physical therapy, cast immobilization, and even surgery may be necessary. Usually you need either to provide more support to the arch or lessen the amount of over-pronation. An arch support or arch pad can provide pain relief. Motion-control shoes can help if you over-pronate.

Stretching can be easily done by bending the knee with the ankle flexed back towards you and gently pulling your toes back towards your knee. Hold this pull to a count of ten and repeat six to ten times a day. Either rolling a tennis ball back and forth under the arch of the foot or simple self-massage across and along the arch also helps. Ice massage can be done using a small frozen juice can rolled under your arch after a run. Orthotics often will help relieve plantar fascia pain. AliMed Rehab and Apex make orthotics for plantar fasciitis. Because self taping of one's arch is difficult, an arch brace is an easy alternative. Providing support to the arch, an arch brace wraps around the arch in order to provide support and decrease the pull of the plantar fascia on the calcaneus heel bone. The Count'R-Force Arch Brace and the PSC wrap are two supports to provide relief from plantar fasciitis pain. The Hapad Longitudinal Metatarsal Arch Pads or 3-Way Heel/Arch/Metatarsal Insoles and the Apex Lynco orthotics may be used to relieve pain.

A lightweight plastic night splint worn to bed can help to stretch the foot and avoid morning stiffness. The night splint helps avoid footdrop and accompanying muscle tightening. Many athletes swear by them. Check with your podiatrist, orthopedist, or medical supply store. AliMed Rehab Products makes several night splints. Lightweight models can easily be carried on a backpack.

Call your podiatrist or orthopedist if you are suffering from pain in the arch of your foot or suspect that you have plantar fasciitis.

An aggressive multi-disciplined medical approach using medical, biomechanical, and physical therapy treatments can help to return you to action as soon as possible.

In an interesting article, "Plantar Fasciitis — A New Perspective", Robert Nirschl, MD, makes a case for plantar fasciitis as a painful degenerative plantar tendinosis, not an inflammation problem.[24] His research found no inflammatory cells in injured plantar fascia which means anti-inflammatory medications and cortisone have no curative potential. For plantar tendinosis Dr. Nirschl recommends stretching and strength training to all areas of the leg to restore strength, endurance, and flexibility. Also recommended is the use of a night splint, arch bracing or a soft orthotic, and footwear with good mid-foot flexibility. In extreme cases, surgery may be indicated to remove painful tendinosis tissue. If your plantar fascia pain does not respond to prescribed treatment, consider asking your podiatrist or orthopedist to look into this study.

Accommodator™ Orthotics   AliMed offers two orthotics to provide relief from plantar fasciitis. The Freedom® Accommodator half-sole orthotic is designed with a contoured heel cup, a shaped longitudinal arch to relieve fatigue while supporting the arch, and a mild metatarsal arch to support and reduce unnecessary pressure from the metatarsal heads. The High-Impact™ Accommodator offers the additional benefit of an Impact Plus™ energy absorbing poromoric polymer pad in the heel. For more information contact AliMed Rehab Products.

Count'R-Force® Arch Brace   Taping of the foot can help but is difficult to do on yourself. The brace is an alternative to taping and is ideal for running and hiking. Designed by an Orthopedic Surgeon/Sports Medicine Specialist, its curved shape allows a wide distribution of the abusive forces causing the pain. Made to fit either foot, an adult universal or small size will fit most individuals. Two tension straps allow for personal adjustment. For more information contact Medical Sports, Inc.

Hapad Arch Pads   Hapad makes several pads which can relieve the discomfort of plantar fasciitis. The Longitudinal Metatarsal Arch Pads provide a corrective action which strengthens the longitudinal and metatarsal arches without restricting the natural flexibility of the foot. Flat feet may also be helped by these pads. The 3-Way Heel/Arch/Metatarsal Insoles is an all-in-one Longitudinal Metatarsal Arch Cushion and heel cushion which relieves plantar fasciitis and foot fatigue by supporting the arch, cushioning the heel and distributing pressure across the ball of the foot. The Comf-Orthotic 3/4-Length Insole is a contoured one-piece arch, metatarsal, and heel cushion which helps support flat feet. The coiled, spring-like wool fibers provide a firm and resilient support as they mold and shape to the foot. For more information contact Hapad, Inc.

Lynco Biomechanical Orthotic Systems   Apex offers the Lynco Biomechanical Orthotic System, a "ready-made" triple-density orthotic system that comes in enough variations to accommodate 90% of foot disorders, including plantar fasciitis. See the chapter *Orthotics* on page 77 for information on these orthotics.

PF™ Night Splint   AliMed Rehab Products makes four models of night splints to relieve the pain of plantar fasciitis. The PF Night Splint is a lightweight plastic splint designed to lessen morning pain caused by contractures and muscle tightening while sleeping. It is set at 5° dorsiflexion (the toes are 5° past 90°). The PF Night Splint II is a deluxe, terry-cloth lined model which adjusts from 10° dorsiflexion to 10° plantar flexion (it comes preset at 5° dorsiflexion). The Early Fit™ Night Splint is fixed at 90° while the Early Fit Adjustable Night Splint can be set from 10° dorsiflexion to 40° plantar flexion. All splints fit both right or left feet and include a liner and straps to protect the leg and instep from pressure. An extra-wide model of the PF Night Splint is offered for those individuals with larger calves and ankles. For more information contact AliMed Rehab Products.

PSC™ by fabrifoam   The PSC is a pronation/spring control device. It is designed to treat plantar fasciitis, chronic heel pain, heel spur syndrome, and shin splints. This reusable strapping device is made from a lightweight, thin foam elastic which breathes and is easily placed on the foot. It wraps around the arch to provide support to the plantar fascia while also wrapping around the heel to reduce the force of heel strike and biomechanically move the foot's mid-line to a more neutral position. For more information contact fabrifoam.

29

Achilles Tendinitis

The Achilles tendon is actually a cord which runs from the calf muscle downward to the back of the heel. The tendon makes it possible for you to rise up on your toes, run, and jump. Achilles tendinitis occurs when the sheath surrounding this cord becomes inflamed. Sudden and repeated stretching of the tendon can cause an inflammation which can produce pain behind the heel, ankle, and lower calf while walking and running. The pain may be felt during the early part of your run or hike, then subside, only to worsen after stopping.

A sudden increase in your mileage or running steep hills can lead to an inflamed Achilles tendon. Increase your mileage gradually or cut down on your hill training.

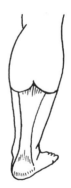

Treatment may include any or all of the following: icing, stretching and flexibility exercises, wearing flexible shoes or boots with a well-padded heel counter, and avoiding the ups and downs of hills. A small heel pad will alleviate the stresses on the tendon. For some individuals, wearing low-heeled shoes as often as possible will help keep the Achilles tendon stretched. An Achilles notch

Achilles tendon

in shoes or mid- and low-top boots will accommodate the Achilles tendon in plantar flexion. If the injury has just happened, use ice packs for the first 48 hours after the injury three to four times a day or until the pain subsides. Thereafter use warm soaks. Stop running — do not run through the pain. Ignoring the symptoms may cause the tendon to rupture, which usually requires surgery. Call your orthopedist or podiatrist if the pain persists. The Achilles Tendon Strap made by Cho-Pat or the Achilles Strap from fabrifoam can provide relief from the discomfort of Achilles tendinitis.

Hapad Heel Pads   Hapad makes the 3/4-Length Heel Wedges which provides necessary heel lift to help reduce the pain associated with Achilles tendinitis. It is available in three thicknesses. The coiled, spring-like wool fibers provide firm and resilient support as they mold and shape to the foot. For more information contact Hapad, Inc.

Achilles Strap by fabrifoam   A new Achilles strap will be released by fabrifoam shortly. For more information contact fabrifoam Products.

Achilles Tendon Strap   Cho-Pat makes this Achilles tendon strap which fits under the arch and around the ankle to relieve pressure on the Achilles tendon. Trials at the Mayo's Sports/ Medicine Clinic have shown the strap effective as an addition to traditional treatment procedures for Achilles tendinitis. The strap is available in four sizes based on ankle circumference at its widest point. It is available by mail order from Cho-Pat, Inc.

30

Metatarsalgia, Morton's Neuroma, and Sesamoiditis

Metatarsalgia is pain somewhere underneath the metatarsal heads of the foot. It typically occurs when one of the metatarsal heads collapses and points downward. Typically the second metatarsal head is affected, but it can also be at the third or fourth heads. It may feel like there is a small stone in your shoe. By pressing up slightly on each metatarsal head you can usually identify the painful area. Usually the metatarsal head which is lower then the others is causing the pain and pressure. There usually will be a callus at the pressure point. A cushioned metatarsal pad can provide relief from metatarsalgia. If the pad does not help, try cutting a small hole in the insole under the painful metatarsal head.

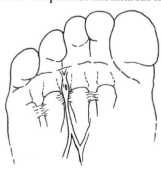

A nerve inflammation indicating Morton's neuroma

Morton's Neuroma is pain associated with a nerve inflammation usually affecting the third and fourth toes. The nerves running between the toes or their sheath has become inflamed and irritated. There is typically tingling, burning, or a pins-and-needles sensation that radiates to the end of the toes. If untreated, scar tissue forms around the nerve and it becomes more painful. The pain is usually relieved by removing the shoe and massaging the foot. If you over-pronate, the metatarsal bones have more movement which can irritate the nerves running between the metatarsal heads. In this case, wearing firm motion-control shoes may help.

Treatments include applying ice to the pain area, an injection of anti-inflammatory medication, wider shoes, a more cushioned insole, and metatarsal pads which take pressure off the metatarsal heads. In some cases surgery may be indicated. Metatarsal pain may also be caused by bursitis, bunions, or arthritis. Your podiatrist or orthopedist can help identify the cause of the pain and make recommendations on how to treat the problems.

Toe exercises help to strengthen and tighten the metatarsal arch and stretch the tendons on top of the toes. Practice picking up marbles with your toes. Put a towel on the floor and use your toes to scrunch up the towel and pick it up.

Sesamoiditis is an inflammation of the two little bones beneath the ball of the foot, under the joint that moves the big toe. These two sesamoid bones can become bruised and inflamed, resulting in sharp pain. The use of soft pads or insoles can help. You can also cut a small hole in your insole under the sesamoid bones.

Hapad Pads Hapad makes several pads to use for these problems. Metatarsal Pads relieve the pain of metatarsalgia and Morton's neuroma. Metatarsal Bars relieve pressure on the ball of the foot that causes painful calluses and forefoot irritations. Metatarsal Cookies provide simple metatarsal arch cushioning. Dancer Pads fit under the ball of the foot with a cutout encompassing the big toe joint to relieve calluses and painful irritations. The coiled, spring-like wool fibers provide firm and resilient support as they mold and shape to the foot. For more information contact Hapad, Inc.

31

Corns, Calluses, and Bunions

A corn is the thickening of the skin, generally on or between the toes, usually caused by friction. Corns on the outer surface of the toes are usually hard while those between the toes are usually soft. To relieve the discomfort of corns, try corn pads, small pieces of one of the tapes mentioned, or Spenco 2nd Skin.

A callus is the thickening of the skin caused by recurring friction, usually on the sole of the foot, most often on the heels or the balls of the feet. A cushioned insole can help equalize the weight load of the foot while pads around or near the callus can relieve pressure. To relieve heel discomfort, try a heel cup or heel pad which will distribute body weight evenly across the heel. Soaking the foot in hot water to soften the callus will allow some of the dead skin to be rubbed off with a callus file or pumice stone.

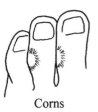

Corns

Warm water soaks and creams or lotions can help soften corns and calluses. See the chapter *Nutrition for the Feet* on page 79 for creams and lotions that can help. Avon makes a foot file described below for use on feet. Geraldine Wales has a

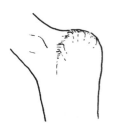

Calluses on
the heel

tendency to get tough calluses on her feet which turn into hot spots and eventually blisters. In the evening she uses the file on the calluses and then applies moisturizing cream to keep her feet soft. Never cut into either corns or calluses with sharp objects.

While there are over-the-counter plantar wart removal compounds available which can also be used on corns and calluses, care must be taken in their use. Common products include DuoFilm® Patch System Wart Removal and Wart-Off® Wart Removal. These products contain salicylic acid. Follow the product's directions to avoid damaging good tissue. Do not use theses products if you are a diabetic. Check your local drug store or pharmacy for a complete line of products.

A bunion is a bump caused by an enlarged bone at the outer base of the big toe where the joint angles inward toward the other toes. Bunions at the outer base of the fifth toe are called bunionettes. The motion of the joint and shoe pressure can cause pain. Be sure your shoes are not too tight. If you over-pronate, try an arch support or orthotic to reduce the over-pronation. Bunion discomfort may be relieved with wider shoes, pads between the big and first toes, arch supports, and warm soaks. Surgery may be necessary in extreme cases.

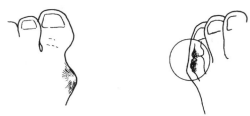

Bunion at the base of the big toe and bunionette on the little toe

A full service shoe shop or a pedorthist should be able to modify a boot to soften a pressure point or stretch a portion of the leather. This may relieve pressure on corns, calluses, and bunions.

Avon's Double Action Foot File   This foot file is 7″ long and has a coarse side and a fine side to remove dry skin buildup and calluses. It can be used on either wet or dry skin. After filing, apply a moisturizing cream. Contact your local Avon sales representative for the file.

Hapad Pads Hapad makes several pads to use for these problems. Metatarsal Pads and Metatarsal Bars reduce pressure on the ball of the foot that causes painful calluses. Metatarsal Cookies provide simple metatarsal arch cushioning which can relieve the pressure which causes corns and calluses. Dancer Pads have a cut out encompassing the big toe joint to relieve calluses and painful irritations. Heel Cushions and Horseshoe Heel Cushions provide comfort from heel calluses. The coiled, spring-like wool fibers provide firm and resilient support as they mold and shape to the foot. For more information contact Hapad, Inc.

32

Athlete's Foot

The hot weather and foot perspiration which runners and hikers typically encounter can make athlete's foot a common problem. The combination of a warm and humid environment in the shoes or boots, excessive foot perspiration, and changes in the condition of the skin combine to create a setting for the fungi of athlete's foot to begin. Athlete's foot usually occurs between the toes or under the arch of the foot. Typical signs and symptoms of athlete's foot include itching, dry skin, cracking, burning, and pain. Left untreated, blisters and swelling may develop.

Treatment includes keeping the feet clean and dry, frequent socks changes, anti-fungal medications, and foot powders. The chapter *Powders* on page 57 has more information on choosing a foot powder. Anti-perspirants may also help those with excessive foot moisture. The chapter *Anti-Perspirants for the Feet* on page 83 has more information about these products. If you use a communal shower or bathrooms after an event, or use a gym to train, avoid walking barefoot in these areas. Use thongs, shower booties, or even your shoes or boots. Check your local drug store or pharmacy for a complete line of athlete's foot anti-fungal ointments, creams, liquids, powders, and sprays. Difficult cases which do not respond to treatment should be seen by a doctor.

If you have a fungal infection of the toenails, check with your local pharmacist for recommended medications. If it does not respond to treatment, a visit to your podiatrist may be necessary.

33

Plantar Warts

Plantar warts occasionally rear their ugly heads and cause foot pain. Usually painful from the pressure of standing and walking, plantar warts can become more painful due to running and hiking. These warts are typically small, hard, granulated lumps on the skin that can be flesh-colored, white, or pink. They are typically found on the bottom of the feet. Plantar warts are caused by a virus that gets into the skin. Moist cracked skin and open or healing blisters leave one susceptible to the virus. Most warts disappear without treatment in four to five months.

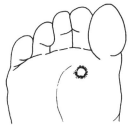

Plantar wart on the ball of the foot

While there are over-the-counter plantar wart removal compounds available, care must be taken in their use. Common products include DuoPlant® Plantar Wart Remover, DuoFilm Patch System Wart Removal, and Wart-Off Wart Removal. These products contain salicylic acid. Follow the product's directions to avoid damaging good tissue. Do not use these products if you are a diabetic. Check your local drug store or pharmacy for a complete line of products. The common medical treatment by podiatrists for plantar warts involves the use of liquid nitrogen to freeze off the wart.

The treatments will put running or hiking on hold until after the spot heals, generally in about a week. Other treatment options include electrical burning, minor surgery, or laser surgery. Check with your podiatrist to determine your treatment options.

34

Foot Care Kits

If you are a runner who finds himself or herself continuously bothered by foot problems, and who often runs long distances without crew support, consider making a small foot care kit to carry in a fanny pack. Hikers should carry a kit, as part of a larger overall first-aid kit, because of their remoteness from assistance. The following items are recommended.

☞ tincture of benzoin swabsticks or squeeze vials

☞ alcohol wipe packets

☞ a pin and matches for blister puncturing

☞ foot powder in a 35mm film canister (with a salt shaker top found at backpacking stores)

☞ a small container for your choice of a lubricant

☞ your choice of tapes wrapped around a pencil

☞ a plastic bag with your choice of blister materials and several pieces of toilet paper or tissues

☞ a small pocket knife with a built-in scissors

You may consider other options to include in the kit, based on your personal foot problems or injury history.

☞ a lightweight ankle support

☞ pads for metatarsal, arch, or heel pain

☞ a heel cup

You can make your own blister kit as described above or purchase a general first-aid kit or a blister medical kit. Most general first-aid kits contain items for basic first-aid care and can be used for blister care by adding a few more specific items. The kits mentioned below are made specifically for blister care. No matter what each kit contains, you should customize the kit to suit your needs and stock it with sufficient equipment for your outing.

Blister Fighter Medical Kit   Outdoor Research offers an 11-ounce Blister Fighter Medical Kit which can be carried in a backpack or kept in a gear bag. The kit contains moleskin, tape, bandages, 2nd Skin pads, Poron donuts, bandage scissors, a razor blade, needles, antibacterial towelettes, benzoin, antibiotic ointment, foot powder, a zip-top bag, and a *Blister Fighter Guide* booklet. The kit comes in a zippered nylon pouch. Contact Outdoor Research for information on ordering the kit.

Mueller Blister Kit   The Blister Kit contains three hydrogel pads, three providone-iodine wipes, and mesh tape for securing the pads. Look for this kit in backpacking or sporting goods stores or contact Mueller Sports Medicine, Inc.

Spenco Blister Kit   This Blister Kit contains four each 2nd Skin pads, adhesive knit strips, and pressure pad ovals. The kit comes in a resealable pouch. Look for this kit in backpacking or sporting goods stores or contact Spenco Medical Corporation.

Part Four

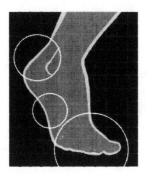

Sources and Resources

35

Medical Specialists

American Academy of Podiatric Sports Medicine
(800) 438-3355
http://www.clark.net/pub/aapsm/aapsm.html
Referrals for podiatrists

American Academy of Orthopaedic Surgeons
(800) 346-AAOS
http://www.aaos.org
Referrals for orthopedic surgeons

American Orthopaedic Foot and Ankle Society
1216 Pine Street, Suite 201, Seattle, WA 98101
(800) 235-4855
http://www.aofas.org
Publications (available by sending a self-addressed
stamped envelope):
> *The Adult Foot*
> *The Ten Points of Proper Shoe Fit*
> *How to Select Sports Shoes*

36

Shoe Review and Gear Review Sources

Backpacker magazine
Rodale Press, Inc., 33 E. Minor Street, Emmaus, PA 18098
Customer Service Department: (800) 666-3434
http://www.bpbasecamp.com
The March issue is their Annual Gear Guide which reviews boots.

Outside magazine
400 Market St., Santa Fe, NM 87501
Customer Service Department: (800) 678-1131
http://outside.starwave.com
The Buyer's Guide is a special magazine typically issued in May.

Runner's World magazine
Rodale Press, Inc., 33 E. Minor Street, Emmaus, PA 18098
Customer Service Department: (800) 666-2828
http://www.runnersworld.com
The April and October issues usually have shoe reviews.

Running Times magazine
Fitness Publishing, Inc., 98 N. Washington St., Boston, MA 02114
Subscriptions & inquiries: (800) 816-4735
The March and September issues usually have shoe reviews.

Ultrarunning magazine
PO Box 2120
Amherst, MA 01004-2120
(413) 584-2640
http://www.ultrarunning.com
Occasional gear reviews and articles with personal experiences
and tips.

37

Product Sources

There are many products mentioned in this book. For each product, the company name, address, telephone number, and Internet address (if available), is provided. Some companies may not sell retail but should be able to identify a local distributor.

Your first source for most of these products should be your local stores. Ask at your running store, backpacking or camping store, pharmacy or drug store, medical supply store, or orthopedic supply store for the products mentioned. While they may not stock all the products mentioned, they may be willing to place a special order.

You may find products similar to those mentioned which are only available in your area. Watching other runners or hikers will often lead to new products they have found to be useful in their foot care efforts. Do not hesitate to ask questions when you see new products.

Rather than use this book as a definitive source, use it as a guide to the wide variety of foot care products available. New products are always being developed. Remember too, your local stores are an excellent source for what is current in the footcare marketplace.

Please be aware that not all companies sell retail and therefore their products may have to be ordered through a store, pharmacy or drug store, podiatrist or orthopedist, or a medical supply or orthopedic supply dealer. Please respect their sales policies.

AA-R Hosiery, PO Box 1118, Elon College, NC 27244
　　Runique™ double layer socks
Acorn, 2 Cedar Street, Lewiston, ME 04243; (800) USA-CORN
　　Fleece socks
AliMed Rehab Products, 297 High Street, Dedham, MA 02026-
9135; (800) 225-2610; http://www.alimed.com
　　PF™ Night Splints and the Accommodator™ orthotics
Allor Medical, Inc., 109 White Oak Lane #92, Old Bridge, NJ
08857; (800) 444-TULI
　　Tuli's® Heel Cups and Coilers™ shoelaces
Apex Foot Health Industries, Inc., 170 Wesley Street, So.
Hackensack, NJ 07606; (800) 526-APEX
　　Lynco® Biomechanical Orthotic Systems
Autumn Harp, 61 Pine Street, Bristol, Vermont 05443; (802)
453-4807
　　Un-Petroleum® Jelly
Avon Products, 9 West 57th Street, NY, NY 10019; (800) FOR-
AVON
　　Silicone Glove creme and Double Action Foot File. Avon
　　products are sold through local sales representatives found
　　in your telephone book.
BodyGlide, 11726 San Vicente Blvd, Suite 220, Los Angeles, CA
90049; (888) 263-9454
　　BodyGlide™ lubricant
Bridgedale Limited, Donaghade Rd., Newtonards, Northern
Ireland BT23 3QR
　　Socks, some with wicking Coolmax
Brown Medical Industries, 481 S. 8th Ave. East, Hartley, IA
51346; (800) 843-4395; http://www.mednetamerica.com/brown
　　Heel Hugger™ and Perform 8™ Lateral Ankle Stabilizer
Bruder Healthcare Company, 1395 S. Marietta Parkway,
Building 630, Marietta, GA 30067; (800) 654-6558;
http://www.bruder.com (Internet site pending)
　　Compeed® blister protection pads
Cho-Pat, Inc., PO Box 293, Hainesport, NJ 08036; (800) 221-
1601; http://www.cho-pat.com
　　Ankle Support, Achilles Tendon Strap, Knee Strap

C & M Pharmacal, Inc., 1721 Maplelane Avenue, Hazel Park, MI 48030; (800) GLYTONE

Hydropel Protective Silicone Ointment (Protective Barrier Ointment)

Cramer Products, Inc., PO Box 1001, Gardner, KS 66030; (800) 255-6621; http://www.cramersportsmed.com

Skin-Lube®, Tuf-Skin®, neoprene ankle support, heel cup: supplied through area distributors

Cropper Medical, 240 East Hersey Street, Ashland, OR 97520; (800) 541-2455

Bio Skin™ ankle and other orthopedic supports

Dahlgren Footwear Inc., PO Box 660614, Arcadia, CA 91066; (800) 635-8539

Dri-Stride® socks with their Climate Knit™ system

Dairy Association Co., Inc., PO Box 145, Lyndonville, VT 05851; (802) 626-3610

Bag Balm salve and lubricant: East of the Rockies

Duke Designs Inc., PO Box 1143, 40500 Downhill Drive, Steamboat Springs, CO 80477; (970) 879-2913

Smartwool™ socks

Dupont, c/o GS&F, 1002 Industrial Road, Old Hickory, TN 37138-3693; (800) 868-2629; http://www.dupont.com/corp/products/prod1021.html

SealSkinz® Waterproof MVT Socks

fabrifoam Products, 900 Springdale Drive, Exton, PA 19341; (800) 577-1077

The PSC™ Pronation/Spring Control device and Achilles Tendinitis strap

Fox River Mills Inc., PO Box 298, Osage, IA 50461; (888) 288-2431

Socks with the Wick Dry® system

Gordon Laboratories, 6801 Ludlow Street, Upper Darby, PA 19082; (800) 356-7870

Gordon's #5, Bromi-Talc and Bromi-Talc Plus powders: through pharmacies only

Hapad, Inc., PO Box 6, 5301 Enterprise Blvd., Bethel Park, PA 15102; (800) 544-2723

Hapad wool felt orthopedic foot products: Longitudinal

Metatarsal, Scaphoid Pads, Metatarsal Pads and Bars, Heel Cushions and Wedges Pads, and Comf-Orthotic® Insoles.

Home Health, 949 Seahawk Circle, Virginia Beach, VA 23452; (800) 284-9123

Podiatrist's Secret™ Total Foot Recovery cream/lotion and Callus Treatment Cream

IMPLUS Corporation, 4900 Prospectus Drive, Suite 300, Durham, NC 27713

Insoles

InterLace Corporation, PO Box 1329, Leominster, MA 01453; (508) 422-6500; http://www.america.com/interlace

Interlace® shoe laces

Kaye & Co. - Easy Laces, PO Box 6261, Sun Valley, ID 83354; (800) 597-2080

Willy's Easy Laces shoe laces

Medical Sports, Inc., Box 7187, Arlington, VA 22207; (800) 783-2240

Count'R-Force® Arch Brace

Medtech Laboratories Inc., PO Box 1683, Jackson, WY 83001; (800) 443-4908

New-Skin® Liquid Bandage

Mueller Sports Medicine, Inc., One French Drive, Prairie du Sac, WI 53578; (800) 356-9522

Runner's Lube, Tuffner Clear Spray, More Skin Pads, Dermal Pads, Blister Kits, neoprene ankle support, and Tuli's Heel Cup™: sells only through distributors

Norm Klein, 11139 Mace River Court, Rancho Cordova, CA 95670; http://www.ultracch.com/html/west_states_100.htm

Gaiters for running shoes and low top hiking boots

Onox, Inc., 43132 Christy Street, Fremont, CA 94538; (800) 533-6669

Foot Solution, Clean-Off, and Itch-Off

Orthopedic Product Sales, 975 Old Henderson, Columbus, OH 43220; (800) 992-9999

Spur Relief Heel Cup: sells only through distributors

Outdoor Research, 2203 1st Avenue South, Seattle, WA 98134-1424; (888) 4OR-GEAR; http://www.orgear.com

Gaiters for running shoes and hiking boots and the Blister Fighter Medical Kit

Patagonia Inc.; 800-336-9090

Socks made with wicking Capilene®

PolyMedica Healthcare, Inc., 581 Conference Place, Golden, CO 80401; (800) 521-4503

Spyroflex® blister protection pads

REI, 1700 45th Street East, Sumner, WA 98390; (800) 426-4840; http://www.rei.com

Outdoor clothes, shoes, boots, and equipment

Seirus Innovative Accessories, 9076 Carroll Way, San Diego, CA 92121; (800) 447-3787

StormSock™ and Neo-Sock®

Smartwool; (800) 550-9665

Merino wool socks

Smith Sales Service, 16372 SW 72nd Avenue, Portland, OR 97223; (503) 639-5479

Bag Balm salve and lubricant: West of the Rockies

Spectrum Sports, Twinsburg, OH 44087

Insoles

Spenco Medical Corporation, PO Box 2501, Waco, TX 76702-2501; (800) 877-3626; http://www.spenco.com

Spenco® 2nd Skin®, Adhesive Knit, Pressure Pads, Insoles and arch supports, Fiberflex™ ankle wrap, and heel pads

Sport Slick Products, 8930 Sepulveda Blvd, #206, Los Angeles, CA 90045-3606; (800) 646-8448

Sport Slick lubricant

Sportsloob, PO Box 16693, Irvine, CA 92713-6693; (800) 525-LOOB

Sportsloob™ lubricant

Stiefel Laboratories, Inc., 255 Alhambra Circle, Coral Gables, FL 33134-7412; (305) 443-3800

Zeasorb® and ZeasorbAF® foot powders

Stromgren Supports Inc., PO Box 1230, Hayes, KS 67601; (913) 625-9036

Double strap ankle support

Superfeet Worldwide LLC, 1419 Whitehorn St., Ferndale, WA 98248; (800) 634-6618; http://www.superfeet.com
> Insoles

Tecnol Consumer Products, 6625 Industrial Park Boulevard, Fort Worth, TX 76180; (800) 832-3182
> Kallassy Ankle Support® — sold retail through Rebound Orthopedic Supports

Thorlo Inc., PO Box 5399, Statesville, NC 28687-5399; (800) 438-0286
> Socks with the Thorlo® System Fit™

Trail Gators, 303 N. Mayflower Avenue, Monrovia, CA 91016; (818) 303-6080
> Trail Gaitors™ for running shoes and low style hiking boots

UCO International, professional reorders only: (800) 541-4030
> Heel Cup 4pf

UltraFit, W5297 Young Road, Eagle, WI 53119; (414) 495-3474
> SUCCEED! Electrolyte Caps

Wigwam Mills Inc., PO Box 818, Sheboygan, WI 53082-0818; (800) 558-7760
> Socks, some with wicking Coolmax®

WrightSock; (800) 654-7191
> Double Layer Socks

Z Knit, Niota, TN 37826
> Polypropylene liner socks

Glossary

Achilles Tendon   The large tendon which runs from the calf to the back of the heel.

Adventure Racing   Multi-sport races over difficult terrain, often done in teams over several days.

Arch   The curved part of the bottom of the foot.

Athlete's Foot   Itchy, red, soggy, flaking and cracking skin between the toes or fluid-filled bumps on the sides or sole of the foot caused by a fungal infection.

Biomechanics   The study of the mechanics of a living body, especially of the forces exerted by muscles and gravity on the skeletal structure.

Blister   A sac between layer of skin filled with fluid which occurs as a result of friction.

Bone Spur   A small bony growth usually indicating a bone irritation.

Bruise   An injury in which blood vessels beneath the skin are broken and blood escapes to produce a discolored area.

Bunion   A bony protrusion at the base of the big toe.

Bunionette   A bunion on the small toe.

Calcaneous   The large heel bone.

Calluses   The thickening of skin caused by recurring friction, usually on the sole of the foot, the heel, or the inner big toe.

Contusion   A bruising injury that does not involve a break in the skin.

Corns	Thickening of the skin, generally on or between the toes, usually caused by friction.

Dermis	The sensitive connective tissue layer of the skin located below the epidermis, containing nerve endings, sweat and sebaceous glands, and blood and lymph vessels.

Edema	Swelling of body tissues due to excessive fluid.

Epidermis	The outer, protective, nonvascular layer of the skin covering the dermis.

Eversion	Movement of the outside of the foot upward as the foot rolls to the inside.

Fibula	The outer and smaller of the two bones of the lower leg.

Flat Foot	A foot that has either a low arch or no arch.

Forefoot	The ball of the foot and the toes.

Heel Pad	The soft tissue pad on the bottom of the heel.

Heel Spur	A small edge of bone which juts out of the calcaneous.

Hematoma	A swelling that contains blood beneath the skin due to an injury to a blood vessel.

Hot Spot	A hot and reddened area of skin that has been irritated by friction.

Hyperhidrosis	Excessive moisture.

Infection	Condition in which a part of the body is invaded by a microorganism such as a bacteria or virus.

Inversion	Movement of the inside of the foot upward as the foot rolls to the outside.

Last	The form over which a shoe or boot is constructed.

Lateral	The outside of the foot, leg, or body.

Ligaments	Strong fibrous connective tissue at a joint that connects one bone to another bone.

Maceration	A breaking down or softening of skin tissue by extended exposure to moisture.

Medial	The inside of the foot, leg, or body.

Metatarsalgia	Pain somewhere underneath the metatarsal heads of the foot.

Midfoot   The mid or center part of the foot containing the arch and five metatarsal bones.

Morton's Neuroma   Pain on the bottom of the foot, usually under the pad of the third or fourth toe.

Morton's Foot   A foot type where the second toe is longer than the big toe.

Neuroma   The swelling of a nerve due to an inflammation of the nerve or the tissue surrounding the nerve.

Orthopedist   An orthopedic surgeon specializing in the treatment and surgery of bones and joint injuries, diseases, and problems.

Orthotics   A molded insert made from a mold of the bottom of the foot which is then inserted into a shoe or boot to correct a foot abnormality.

Pedorthist   A specialist trained to work on the fit or modification of shoes and orthotics to alleviate foot problems caused by disease, overuse, or injury.

Plantar Fascia   The band of fibers along the arch of the foot which connects the heel to the toes.

Plantar Fasciitis   An inflammation of the plantar fascia.

Plantar Warts   Small, hard, flesh colored, white, or pink granulated lumps typically found on the feet and caused by a virus.

Podiatrist   A doctor of podiatric medicine who specializes in the treatment and surgery of the foot and ankle.

Pronation   An abnormal rolling over of the foot towards the inside of the body when weight bearing.

RICE   The acronym for rest, ice, compression and elevation, which are used for sprain and strain injuries.

Sesamoiditis   An inflammation of the two little bones beneath the ball of the foot, under the joint that moves the big toe.

Sole   The bottom of the foot.

Sprain   A joint injury in which ligament damage is sustained.

Sterilization   The process of the removal of bacteria.

Strain   Muscular injury produced by overuse or abuse of a muscle.

Subungal Hematoma   A hemotoma under the nail plate.

Supination The rolling of the foot towards the outside of the body when weight bearing.

Tendinitis An inflammation of a tendon or its surrounding sheath.

Tendons The elastic tough fibrous tissue that connects muscles to bone.

Toe Box The front part of a shoe or boot that covers the toes.

Ultrarunning Running distances greater than a marathon.

Virus A tiny organism that causes disease.

Wart A thickened, painful area of skin caused by a virus.

Endnotes

[1]   J.J. Knapik, K.I. Reynolds, K.L. Duplantis, and B.H. Jones. "Friction Blisters: Pathophysiology, Prevention and Treatment." *Sports Medicine* (20 (3) 1995), p. 140.

[2]   12 miles per day times, 5,280 feet/mile divided by 2.5 feet/step. For each mile more than 12 add 2100 steps. For each mile less than 12 subtract 2100 steps.

[3]   Ray Jardine, *The Pacific Crest Trail Hiker's Handbook* (LaPine, OR: Adventure Lore Press, 1996), p. 93.

[4]   The usual issues are: *Backpacking* (March is the Annual Gear Guide Issue), *Outside* (May Buyer's Guide), *Runner's World* (April and September), and *Running Times* (March and September).

[5]   J.D. Denton, Dennis Grandy, D.P.M., and Tom Kennedy, "How to Find the Right Shoe for You" *Running Times* (September 1996), p. 16, and "How to Find a Shoe That Works." *Running Times* (March 1997), p. 18.

[6]   Tom Brunick, and Bob Wischnia, "Choosing the Right Shoe" and "Know Your Foot Type." *Runner's World* (April 1997), p. 52.

[7]   J.J. Knapik, K.L. Reynolds, K.L. Duplantis, and B.H. Jones, "Friction Blisters: Pathophysiology, Prevention and Treatment." *Sports Medicine* (20 (3) 1995), p. 142.

[8]   Tim Noakes, MD, *The Lore of Running* (Champaign, IL: Leisure Press, 1991), p. 460.

[9] Robert Boeder, *Beyond the Marathon: The Grand Slam of Trail Ultrarunning* (Vienna, GA: Old Mountain Press, 1996), p. 22.

[10] J.J. Knapik, K.L. Reynolds, K.L. Duplantis, and B.H. Jones, "Friction Blisters: Pathophysiology, Prevention and Treatment." *Sports Medicine* (20 (3) 1995), p. 139.

[11] Andrew Lovy, "New Blister Formula Revealed! Free!" *Ultrarunning* (April 1990), p. 40.

[12] Colin Fletcher, *The Complete Walker III* (New York: Alfred A. Knopf, 1996), p. 86.

[13] Richard Benyo, *The Death Valley 300: Near-Death and Resurrection on the World's Toughest Endurance Course* (Forestville: Specific Publications, 1991), p. 142.

[14] Gary Cantrell, "From the South: The Amazing Miracle of Duct Tape." *Ultrarunning* (December, 1988), p. 36-37.

[15] Donald Baxter, MD; David Porter, MD, Ph.D.; Paul Flahavan, C.Ped; and Charles May, "The Ideal Running Orthosis: A Philosophy of Design." *Biomechanics* (March, 1996), p. 41-44.

[16] Tim Noakes, MD, *The Lore of Running* (Champaign, IL: Leisure Press, 1991), p. 459.

[17] J.J. Knapik, K.L. Reynolds, K.L. Duplantis, and B.H. Jones, "Friction Blisters: Pathophysiology, Prevention and Treatment." *Sports Medicine* (20 (3) 1995), p. 138.

[18] Ibid., p. 140.

[19] Ibid., p. 139.

[20] Bryan Bergeron, MD, "A Guide to Blister Management." *The Physician and Sportsmedicine* (February 1995), p. 40.

[21] Ibid., p. 43.

[22] William Trolan, MD, *Blister Fighter Guide* (Seattle: Outdoor Research 1996).

[23] "The Conservative Treatment of Plantar Fasciitis; A Prospective Randomized, Multicenter Outcome Study" (American Orthopaedic Foot and Ankle Society, October 1996).

[24] Robert Nirschl, MD. MS, "Plantar Fasciitis — A New Perspective." *American Medical Joggers Association AMAA Quarterly.* (Summer 1996).

Bibliography

Ellis, Joe, D.P.M. with Joe Henderson. *Running Injury-Free.* Emmaus, PA: Rodale Press, 1994.

Jardine, Ray. *The Pacific Crest Trail Hiker's Handbook.* LaPine, OR: AdventureLore Press, 1996.

McGann Daniel M, D.P.M. and L. R. Robinson. *The Doctor's Sore Foot Book.* New York: William Morrow and Company, Inc., 1991.

Noakes, Tim, MD. *The Lore of Running.* Champaign, IL: Leisure Press, 1991.

Schneider, Myles J., D.P.M. and Mark D. Sussman, D.P.M. *How to Doctor Your Feet Without a Doctor.* Washington, D.C.: Acropolis Books, Ltd., 1984.

Subotnick, Steven I., D.P.M., M.S. *The Running Foot Doctor.* San Francisco: World Publications, 1977.
——, *Sports & Exercise Injuries: Conventional, Homeopathic, & Alternative Treatments.* Berkeley: North Atlantic Books, 1991.

Tremain, David M., MD and Elias M. Awad, Ph.D. *The Foot & Ankle Sourcebook.* Los Angeles: Lowell House, 1996.

Trolan, William, MD. *Blister Fighter Guide*. Seattle: Outdoor Research, 1996.

Weisenfeld, Murry F., MD with Barbara Burr. *The Runner's Repair Manual*. New York: St. Martin's Press, 1980.

About the Author

John Vonhof brings a varied background and extensive experience to *Fixing Your Feet*. This book, which he wrote and illustrated, is the synthesis of over 15 years of experience as a runner and hiker.

Having run since 1982, John discovered the challenging world of trail running and ultras in 1984. Over the years, he has completed more than 20 ultras: 50 kms, 50 milers, 100 milers, 24-hour runs, and a 72-hour run. John has completed the difficult Western States 100 Mile Endurance Run three times and the Santa Rosa 24-Hour Track Run ten times.

In 1987 John, with fellow runner Will Uher, fastpacked the 211 mile John Muir Trail in the California High Sierra's in 8.5 days with 30 pound packs. A solo repeat trip is planned for the fall of 1997. In between have been shorter backpacking trips.

As race director of the Ohlone Wilderness 50 KM Trail Run for the past ten years, John has worked at providing a quality event for runners of all skill levels. This run is known as one of the most difficult 50 km trail ultras in Northern California.

An opportunity to change careers in 1992 led him into the medical field where he now works as an emergency room technician with certifications as a paramedic and orthopedic technician. Over the years he has provided volunteer medical aid at numerous running events.

This background has provided a wealth of learning opportunities for what can go wrong with feet and ways to fix them.

Index

A

Accommodator Orthotics 139
Achilles tendinitis 141
Achilles Tendon Strap 142
ACORN socks 49, 50, 54
Adhesive felt 110
Advanced blister care 111
Adventure racing 9
Alignment, of the body 14
American Academy of Orthopaedic Surgeons 8, 31, 157
American Academy of Podiatric Sports Medicine 8, 157
American Orthopaedic Foot and Ankle Society 8, 157
Andrew Lovy's lubricant formula 60
Ankle supports 124
Anti-perspirants for the feet 83
Arch 14
Asphalt, running on 17
Athlete's Foot 148
Avon
   Double Action Foot File 146
   Silicone Glove lubricant 60

B

Backpacker magazine 159
Bag Balm lubricant 60

I

K

L

M

N